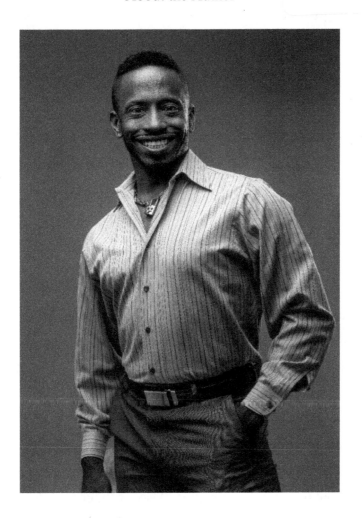

Photo by Don Harris © Don Harris Photographics, LLC. All rights reserved

Justin Terry-Smith was born in Columbia Maryland and was raised in the suburbs of Washington DC (Silver Spring, Maryland). He graduated from Paint Branch High School in 1998. He joined the United States Air Force in 1999 and was discharged honorably with awards and decorations in 2003. Justin moved back to the DC area and began to work for a DC HIV Non-profit. After 3 years of working in the HIV community, he himself was diagnosed with HIV. He did not let that stop him from living life. He eventually went back to college and earned an Associates in Communications from Axia College, a Bachelors in Political Science from Ashford University, and a Masters and Doctorate in Public Health from Walden University. He has been married since 2009 and has two sons, Lundyn and Tavis. Justin is of African American and Jewish descent/ancestry. In his spare time, he is pursuing acting and philanthropic avenues. The Advice in this book is the same advice Justin has given to his readers in the magazine A&U Magazine.

Just*in Time: February 2012

February 21, 2012

by Justin B. Terry-Smith

Hi Justin,

I was just wondering what your view was on abstinence? Do you think it is a good thing, possible, or is it unrealistic?

Thanks in advance.—gypsykatcher30

Gypsy,

Every time I hear one of my friends say, "I'm going to be abstinent," I think about the reasons why they might say so. There are so many reasons. Some of the people I know decide to because of spiritual reasons, some do it because they are scared of catching HIV or an STI, and others because they suffer from low self-esteem and fear rejection. Listen, if you want to remain abstinent it is okay. I honestly think that anyone who wants to can but do it for the right reasons. Do it because you want to and not because you are scared of something. Most of the friends that I have that are abstinent for spiritual reasons usually are able to be abstinent longer than my friends that do not, but that is only my experience. Also, abstinence is the only 100 percent way not to be sexually infected with HIV or any other STI. I for one could not do it at all. As some of you know I have been married since August 7, 2009, but before I dated my husband, I was single, and I thought about abstinence. Honey, if it works for you do it, but as for me I could not.

Justin,

I have been seeing a man for about two years now. I have been positive for about five years; my boyfriend is also HIV-positive, and he has been infected since 2006. He wants to have unprotected sex. Should I do it? I am so unsure about this—please help!
—Antonio

Antonio,

Listen up and listen up good. Do not do something you are unsure about or something that you are scared of. Go with your gut. I cannot tell you what to do but I can only speak of what I would do. I have been with the same man for almost six years and we still have protected sex. Just because you both have HIV does not mean that neither one of you are not opened to being able to be infected with other STIs. There are things such as hepatitis C, herpes, chlamydia, gonorrhea, and syphilis, etc., that you can catch without using a condom.

But there is another side of the controversial subject that I will try to explain, because my opinion is not the be-all end-all say-so of sex between two HIV-positive people. So, you and your partner have been together and, if you are monogamous, there are some ways that people can get around harming either HIV-positive partner when having unprotected sex, but they are very risky. You need to have a very open and honest conversation with your partner about STIs, drug resistance, and treatment history. With HIV comes being susceptible to other STIs. Be ready to take those infections on just in case you are infected with one of them. Please keep in mind that chlamydia, gonorrhea, and syphilis are curable and less harmful if caught and treated early, but there is no cure for hepatitis C or herpes.

Knowing your resistances to any HIV drugs is paramount in this context, too. For example, say you are taking Atripla and you become resistant to Atripla; if you have unprotected sex then there is a chance that your partner might become resistant to his own medication. Past treatment is also important as well. Please discuss all the above with your partner. Thanks…and as the fabulous Miranda Priestley from the infamous movie The Devil Wears Prada says, "That's all!"

Just*in Time: March 2012

March 5, 2012

by Justin B. Terry-Smith

**What's up, Justin?**

Listen, I have been reading and watching your blog, Justin's HIV Journal, and I have been a fan of yours and it is truly inspirational to see your strength through it all. Well, all in all, I have been diagnosed with HIV for a year now and I have been very open with my status to guys I have tried to date and to even some of my friends. Now I am single, and I feel more alone than ever. I have tried to date poz guys, but most of the ones I have met want to only bareback and I do not want any part of it. I am scared I will be alone for the rest of my life until the day I die. Any words of advice for me?

—Jason

**Jason,**

Hey, I am sure that some people who are reading your letter and who are HIV-positive will say that they have been there before, and I am not an exception. When I found out that I was HIV-positive, it was not easy dating at all. I had one guy who I was dating that told me he never wanted to see me again. Lo and behold, he also became HIV-positive about two years later.

We have to be strong and know that there will be someone out there that will love us for who we are and not see disease when looking into our eyes or soul. Now, when a man says that he does not want you because of your status, respect his decision and move on. The more time you waste thinking about a person who does not want you, the more time is wasted not looking for the one who does want you.

Look inside yourself and know that you are beautiful inside and out and if someone cannot see that then fuck them.

Also, and this has helped me, I suggest that you find an activity that makes you happier than hell and go for it head-on. Keep in mind, too, that there are groups that do have a poz theme to them that are not about dating but about networking and having people that are or will go through the same things you are. Also, if your friends are starting to turn their backs on you just because you have HIV then they are not really your friends and you do not need that drama.

I find that there are a lot of people who want a relationship when they are first diagnosed because they are looking for that acceptance that it is okay and that someone will love them. I am not saying this is happening with you but keep that in perspective. All I am saying is that be comfortable with yourself and love yourself—then that will open your heart to be loved by someone else.

**Justin,**

I need your help. My boyfriend and I have been together for two months and I really love him. We met at a club in Philadelphia; he was dancing and when I saw him, I was instantly attracted to him. I started to dance with him, and we eventually sat down for a drink and to talk. After that, we started seeing each other sporadically, but recently our relationship has gotten more and more serious. The more we are together the closer we are to having sex. I do not know what to do— should I tell him?
—Michelle

**Michelle,**

Okay, honey, this is a situation that we all as HIV-positive people have to deal with. The "should I tell him or her and how" question is a hard one to swallow. But sweetie, hold on, because you might need some water to swallow it down.

Okay, in my opinion, tell him!!! Well, if you two have not been intimate then that is good because he should at least have the choice of knowing that this is not what he wants. Give him the option to say "no" or to say "yes."

In my opinion, the earlier you tell him the more he will respect you in the end. Also, there are laws in some states that have been enacted to criminalize people who are living with HIV. I am not here to scare you, but you need to know the truth.

When you tell him, I suggest that you do so in a very comfortable and familiar setting to you both. Be very careful. When telling a loved one it can be very hard. I can relate—I did not even get a chance to tell my own mother; she found out through a family member, one I thought I could trust. It is better if he hears from you than one of your friends or family members. Remember, Michelle, there are worse things than to tell your partner that you have HIV, and that would be to not tell him. Stay strong honesty is the best policy.

Just*in Time: April 2012
April 5, 2012

by Justin B. Terry-Smith

Justin,

I found you through a search on Google for HIV. I need your help. I am an HIV-negative female. I have a best friend named David. We have been friends for sixteen years and it was back in high school that we met. We dated briefly but we decided to become friends and plus he was gay—LOL. But the reason why I am writing you is because he found out a couple of months ago that he was HIV-positive. When he told me, I broke down and cried; we cried together for at least an hour. After that he started going out to clubs a lot and stopped calling as often. I visited him and I have never seen his house look so dirty. Dust was everywhere and he looked like hell and obviously was not taking care of himself. I want to know what I should do. Please let me know what you think I should do.
—With + love,
HIV-Negative Woman

Dear HIV-Negative Woman,

Okay, there are so many things that I could tell you. But in my opinion, he sounds like he is depressed. After finding out that I was HIV-positive the same thing happened to me. I started going out without my friends and I started doing a lot of things that I would not normally do. I started partying late, drinking a lot, and doing drugs.

Then I met someone who helped me. He looked at my apartment, looked at me and held me. He told me, "Let it out," and then I cried. Now I am not saying that you should do this with David but what I will say is that, if you really want to help you have to love him, and now that the simple part is out of the way, check him! It is time to not let him get away with anything. Evaluate the situation and try to be there for him. He might want to go into counseling as well. Sometimes we can admit things to strangers more easily than we can admit things to friends and family. HIV is a tough cookie to swallow—when some of us are diagnosed we become instantly depressed and HIV feeds on that depression. We should never go down without a fight. I say this because I most definitely will not, and neither should David. Try to pull him out of his rut. Love him and then show him.

Dear Justin,

I have decided to stop taking my meds. They make me tired all the time and I do not like what they have done to my cholesterol or skin. I have been watching one of your videos on Justin's HIV Journal and I see that you were going through the same thing. Do you have any advice for me?

—Divo

Divo,

You bet I do. This matter I take rather seriously. Take supplements to help level your cholesterol and watch what you eat as it also contributes to skin care as well.

Now, let us talk about you wanting to stop taking your meds. It is your choice but be aware of the consequences. You are going to leave yourself open to more infections because HIV disrupts your immune system and the meds that you are taking are not only helping to stop HIV from becoming unmanageable, but they are also helping your body to keep fighting against other infections. Like cancer. Your body fights off cancer cells every day; when someone has HIV, the body starts concentrating on HIV but has to have enough T-cells to fight against the cancer as well.

Analyze why you wish to stop taking meds. My friend Joshua just died on the 19th of March because he stopped taking his meds. He got sick and he died. His name goes on a list of so many others that I have known, and I am only thirty-two.

All in all, stay on your meds.

Just*in Time: June 2012
June 21, 2012

**Justin,**

**You probably get messages like this a lot, but I am a little worried.**

**I had unprotected sex about six to seven months ago. I was a virgin, and he was, too. He claimed he was "clean" and everything, but my state of mind was not really all that good afterwards.**

**Anyway, I am worried I might have been exposed to HIV, but I have not had any of the symptoms, like lymph nodes swelling, though about two weeks ago I got a cold...well, I hope that it was a cold. My glands did not swell, and I got a sore throat for a bit and I kept having these heat spikes where my temperature would go up and then down, but only lasting a few seconds. I am still sniffling. Toward the end of the major symptoms my gums started to ache, and my jaw hurt, too. I might be worrying over nothing, but I just hope you can give me some advice. I mean if I have it can I still live a long life?**
**—Harvey**

Well, after reading your question I wanted to break it down so I, for one, better understand. Okay, so he said he was a virgin. Ask yourself this, "How can you look at someone and tell they are a virgin?" The answer is you cannot. Also using substances that lower your inhibitions make you more susceptible to HIV/AIDS. So, we must watch out for ourselves and ask questions.

If you are worried that you might have been exposed, then the best thing to do is to get tested for HIV. HIV is a tricky disease, and it is different with everyone. Some people have no symptoms at all, even when they have been infected for a long time. Also, if you are having a sore throat, heat spikes, and other viral symptoms, you might want to see a doctor. The best thing that you could do in either situation—whether it is a common cold or something HIV-related—is to get medical attention. Also, if you are infected with HIV you can still live a long healthy life, but you will have to take care of yourself more than you used to. In a study researcher predicted that a twenty-year-old person starting HIV medications between 1996 and 1999, the early years of combination antiretroviral drug therapy, could expect to live an additional thirty-six years, to the age of fifty-six, than if they were not on treatment. Over time the number of years increased significantly. A twenty-year-old who started treatment between 2003 and 2005 could expect to live an additional forty-nine years, to the age of sixty-nine. Now these numbers are great but make sure that you stick with your medications, exercise, and eat right. You will be okay, negative, or positive. ☺

**Hi Justin,**

**I subscribed to your YouTube channel recently and I absolutely adore your videos. Not only are you incredibly courageous, but you are also so well spoken and intelligent! You emanate strength, and everything that you are doing for the community as a whole is truly remarkable. Praise aside, I do have a question for you: What are your thoughts on the HIV [antibody] testing window period? It is something that truly disturbs me; the thought that I could be positive but test negative regardless is torturous. I have been tested many times in my life, all of which have thankfully come back negative, but I struggle with never having peace of mind. The constant doubt lingers, "Okay, so you're 'negative,' but what if your results were only negative because you were exposed too recently for the test to detect?"**
**—Rebecca**

Yes, I am a big advocate for people knowing their status. The window period is something that we cannot do anything about now. I tell people who are sexually active to get tested every three months. Getting tested every three months can shave down that window a tad. Also, there is even a better test to close that window known as the Architect HIV Ag/Ab combo assay, which can catch the infection early. Studies have shown that this particular test may detect HIV up to twenty days earlier than antibody-only tests, which is important in controlling the spread of the virus.

Just*in Time: July 2012
July 20, 2012

**Justin,**

**I am somewhat of an "AIDS denialist." For all that I have researched, read, studied, and learned, I have a hard time accepting what I've "unlearned." At the same time, the passing of a close cousin and Christine Maggiore has forced me to ask myself, 'If I were HIV-positive, would I have the strength of my convictions to live the life I advocate, like Christine, or would I take the path that most people take?' My mind rejects conventional wisdom on HIV and the use of HIV medications, but I do not think I would take the "holistic" route, either. I just do not understand why there cannot be an alternative clinical**

**option. Let me know what your thoughts are. Thanks!**

**—dnahotep**

Let me just say there are a lot of AIDS or HIV denialists that e-mail me almost daily. What do denialists believe? First, they question whether or not HIV is the cause of AIDS. A lot of denialists do not think that HIV is a sexually transmitted disease. If they are positive, they do not take HIV medications; they also believe that alternative medicines, exercise, vitamins, massage, yoga, and other unproven treatments will stop the progression of the disease. I, too, practice yoga and take vitamins, but I also take my HIV meds. It pains me to see people who deny that HIV exists or that it is easily taken care of by just alternative medicine when most of the public, scientists, and educators know better. Try going to www.aidstruth.org to find a little clarity.

When denialists influence a nation's political figures, it is detrimental to its citizens, even to the point of death. Unfortunately, denialists go to less informed countries to spread their views. Former South African president Thabo Mbeki who was directly influenced by Peter H. Duesberg, a huge AIDS denialist, believed Duesberg and now he is responsible for over 365,000 deaths in South Africa alone. Mbeki also was convinced that Western Civilization blamed Africans for HIV/AIDS; he also tried to tie the early colonialism of Africa to HIV/AIDS.

"Convinced that we are but natural-born, promiscuous carriers of germs, unique in the world, they proclaim that our continent is doomed to an inevitable mortal end because of our unconquerable devotion to the sin of lust," Thabo Mbeki stated. See, ignorance is truly bliss. Even if his theory were true, why didn't he focus on HIV instead of blaming scientists, Western Civilization, racism, etc? That is what denialism does, deny, deny, deny—and then blame. Compare this with the countries in Africa that are confronting HIV and finding infection rates and deaths from HIV going down because they have made HIV education and prevention resources available to their people.

Another example of denialism is Christine Maggiore, who was diagnosed with HIV in 1992. She met with Duesberg who convinced her to think that her positive test may have been due to flu shots, or a common viral infection. Maggiore became pregnant and was told to start HIV medication to help prevent HIV from reaching her unborn child. She refused. Then when the baby was born, she breastfed her newborn, which potentially heightens the chances of infection in babies.

The newborn died of what the coroner called, "Pneumocystis pneumonia in the setting of advanced AIDS." Maggiore would eventually lose her own battle on December 27, 2008, and, yes, I did blog about it.

It is tragic how HIV denialism can misinform people around the world, especially in developing countries. It is because of these misguided souls that we have things like the International AIDS Conference, so that we can have a dialogue and learn more about HIV/AIDS. We need to keep all channels open about these kinds of things so that we may become closer to eradicating this horrific disease.

By the way, the International AIDS Conference will be held in D.C. from July 22–27. This is the first time it has been held in the U.S. in twenty-two years and I hope to see some of you there.

Silence = Death…and so does Denialism.

Just*in Time: August 2012
August 25, 2012

**Hey Justin,**

**I am trying to hang in there but dealing with these meds is quite difficult and sometimes I do not know what to do and [I am] feeling alone. I admire the things you do, and you seem, like many others, to at least enjoy some "normal" quality of life. I feel so drugged in the morning and can hardly get out of bed. Hmm, it is like a nightmare worse than Elm Street. LOL. I see why some people give up on [drug regimens], but it is like being between a rock and a hard place. If you do, it is like hell, and, if you do not, it is probably straight to hell! LOL. (I am trying to make light of my situation.) Anyway, I hope to hear from you and that there might be a bright side. Thanks.**

**—Dwight, Jamaica**

First of all, thank you so much for the compliment. Second, take it easy on yourself—the more stress that you put on yourself the more the virus can disrupt your system and even your way of thinking. I suggest doing something to lower your stress levels. Know that this is just a hill that we, as HIV-positive people, have to climb. No matter what happens, keep a positive mindset.

Third, the medications work with everyone's system a little differently. At first, I was on Truvada, Norvir, and Reyataz. It was fine at first, but then it started making my eyes yellow and my skin got a little darker. It literally gave me jaundice and it hurt my self-esteem as well. The meds do make some of us tired, but you must tell your doctor this. There are some things that your doctor can do to help you in this matter. He or she might put you on a different HIV medication that might help you with your fatigue. Also, what I do is to take vitamins that help me with my energy levels, not to mention my coffee-a-day regimen. LOL. Fourth, do not give up on your medications. I know it seems like they are not helping, but they are. They are making sure that your body keeps the HIV in check. I do not know what medications you are on, but I, too, had the same feeling mentally and physically when I first started on my HIV regimen. Now, about feeling alone. I have to ask if there are any support groups around you in Jamaica. I have found out that having someone near you that might be going through the same things you are does help. You have the ability to reach out to them when you are feeling low or having troubles with the medications that you are on. I think you should do some research on finding a group that does deal with HIV openly and head-on so that you are not susceptible to low self-esteem and are able to take more control over what you might think is uncontrollable—your life.

**Justin,**

**I do not know if I can handle this anymore, but I do not want to take my medications. Each day I get up and wonder if it will be my last. I feel so weak, but some of the government officials in my country have told me that HIV is not a real disease. What should I do? —Abdul, South Africa**

Go see a doctor who has the mentality that HIV is a disease and can be controlled. I do not know if a doctor is available for you to see quickly, but you should do some research and find one. HIV medications have saved many lives, including my own. I had a friend named Joshua who stopped taking his meds. I saw him early this year and he looked a little skinnier and was pale. His family buried him last month. He was an ex-roommate of mine and I loved him dearly. The more we take control of our medical health, the better we are able to combat the disease. I do not know if HIV medications are available to you, but I know that they have made my life worth living—for my husband, my friends, my family and, most of all, me.

Just*in Time: September 2012
September 17, 2012

**Justin, I found your site through a friend of mine who knows you personally, but I do not want to share his name. I am a twenty-six-year-old HIV-positive female. Well, I just found out two days ago that I am pregnant. I am scared of transmitting HIV to my unborn child; what should I do? I have not been to see my regular doctor yet. Please help me. What should I do?—Andrea**

Go see your doctor immediately. Listen, the faster you see a doctor the more that can be done about taking preventive measures to protect your unborn child. Okay, so here are some facts. Yes, a mother can pass on HIV to her unborn child but if precautions are taken this percentage is lowered to single digits. There are HIV medications that many women take during pregnancy. Also, when the child is born, doctors might suggest that he or she start on medications as well. When delivery time is near you could opt for a C-section or vaginal delivery, depending on the state of your health. During childbirth there are a lot of fluids between mother and baby, but the less fluid during the delivery the better. But the main thing is to see a doctor; they will run blood tests on you and be upfront about your HIV status so that they know to take the proper precautions to protect you and your unborn child. When your doctor runs all the blood tests, HIV will come up anyway, whether you tell them or not. Trust and believe that you will be fine. I am not your doctor and I cannot tell you if your child will be born HIV-positive or not but think positively—it is beneficial to your state of mind and your baby. Just keep in mind that you are thinking for two. By the way, congratulations!

**Justin,**
**My wife and I are HIV-positive, and we feel that breastfeeding is a bonding moment for the mother and child. We are not going to breastfeed our baby, who is HIV-negative, because we are afraid that we would pass on HIV to our baby. But we have friends that beg to differ. I think they are more worried about bonding with their child than they are about the health of their own child. I want to ask you your opinion because I know they read your column. They have told us that their child is HIV-negative but continue to breastfeed him. What do you think they should do?—HIV Parents**

Well, let me just say congrats on the baby and I am so happy for you both. I hope your friends are reading this. They need to stop breastfeeding immediately or take proper precautions to lower the infection rate; just because their child is now HIV-negative it does not mean that the child will not develop HIV later on through breastfeeding by the HIV-positive mother. Even though breastfeeding has been proven beneficial to both baby and mother it has a chance of HIV infection. Breast milk is filled with nutrients and antibodies that can protect the child against diseases, but it has never been proven that it protects against HIV. Also, as the baby grows and matures, so does breast milk to better adapt to the baby's needs. The mother while breastfeeding has a lower rate of being diagnosed with certain diseases as well. These benefits are great but, being HIV-positive, one must take precautions. In this area of HIV transmission, breastfeeding, I am afraid, must be avoided. But you can feed your baby in another way, by using commercial formula. In many parts of the world breastfeeding is the only option because of lack of finances and resources. One out of four children worldwide are infected with HIV through breastfeeding. I hope you are listening.

Just*in Time: October 2012

October 3, 2012

by Justin B. Terry-Smith

**Hi Justin,**

**I actually just read on your blog, Justin's HIV Journal, that you are now a foster/adoption parent in the state of Maryland—that is wonderful. [Editor's note: Justin and his husband Phil just became foster/adoptive parents to a beautiful LGBT teen in Maryland.] I am so happy for you both; I know that it is truly a blessing and a joy to add a little one into your life. How old is the child? Did you tell the child about your HIV? If so, how did you do this? The reason why I am asking is because I need to tell my son. He is a very rambunctious, intelligent boy. He is about twelve years old and I really do not know what to say to him. I love my son and I do not want to hurt or scare him in any way. I care for him more than I care about my own life or others around me. His mother died at childbirth and I now have met a woman that I plan on marrying next year. She and I fell in love at first sight and actually met on an HIV-positive dating site.**

**My son means the world to me and I do not know what to say. Please tell me what to do.**
**—Positive Father**

Hey, first off, thank you so much for the compliment. Our son is adorable and very special to us. Already calling us Daddy (me) and Dad (Phil), he made me cry for the first time.

Okay, when we brought him into our lives, we decided to be open and honest with him. You have to understand that if you do not tell children the truth when they ask a question, and if they find out that you have been lying to them, there is a chance they might not ever trust you. We told him the truth and he was okay with it. You have to understand that our child is a teen and yours, I am guessing, is younger. But, with all children just answer their questions as best as you can. Be forward and upfront with your son. Let him know that everything will be okay, and he should not be afraid of you just because you have HIV. I would also do this at a time and place that is familiar to him and to make sure there is nobody else around. Educate him about HIV and reassure him that DADDY WILL BE OK ☺.......AND SO WILL HIS FUTURE MOMMY.

**Hey, Justin!**
**I found your site from my gay cousin, who loves you. Anyways, I was hoping you could help me out with something. My girlfriend is HIV-positive, right? And I am not. Okay, so here it goes. I have had sex with HIV-positive women before and I never seem to catch it. But I heard that you still could catch it—am I just lucky or what?**
**—Juan**

Well, thank your cousin for me for supporting me and my cause. Listen, buddy, and listen well. I do not know how many HIV-positive women that you have slept with without a condom, but all it takes is just one time for you to catch HIV. One time! Sometimes, when someone is exposed to HIV, it could take years for immune system problems to start. Also, there are people on this earth that have had sex with people that are HIV-positive but do not ever get the disease, but that is slim to none.

You need to be careful as well because HIV is not the only STD/STI (sexually transmitted disease/sexually transmitted infection) you can catch. Some consider hepatitis C even worse. There is also syphilis and other diseases for which you would have to be reported to your state health department and, if you do not comply with their requirements, then they come to your house with a car labeled, "STATE HEALTH DEPT." Lovely thought…isn't it?

Just*in Time: November 2012

November 1, 2012

by Justin B. Terry-Smith

**Dear Justin,**

**I have a question: Can openly gay men who are positive join the Army or Air Force?**
**—Detox**

I was in the Air Force for four years. I served honorably as an HIV-negative, semi-closeted gay man. When I say semi-closeted, I mean I did not tell anyone about my sexuality unless they were family or close friends. I had a really good group of friends in the military who were also gay— James, Chris, and Tyler. We all hung out and were there for each other in our darkest hours.

After serving four years I was discharged honorably from the U.S. Air Force, with awards and decorations, and I was very proud to have served my country. After leaving the Air Force I often wondered if I could go back in the military. In 2006 I was diagnosed with HIV but still had that deep question in my mind, "Could I get back into the military even if I were HIV-positive?"

If you are HIV-negative when you started your service in any military branch and you are infected with HIV, they give you an option. The option is: You can leave for medical reasons or you can stay in, but you cannot go overseas to any hazardous zones; rather, you will have to be stationed in the U.S.

When I was stationed at Dover AFB, I met a Navy man who was stationed at the Pentagon. He was so handsome that I really started to like him. We dated for a while and then he decided not to see me anymore. His reason was that he did not want to engage in a long-distance relationship. That man was HIV-positive, and we are still friends to this day. (He is not the one who infected me, just to be clear. We were very careful.) I asked him how he became HIV-positive and he told me that it was a woman overseas who had infected him. The Navy asked whether he wanted to be medically discharged or stay in. He decided to stay in and is retiring very soon.

So, you see you have to be HIV-negative when you enter the military, but you have the option to stay in if you are infected while still in the military. As far as trying to enter the military while being HIV-positive, that is a big negative, Detox. You cannot enter the military if you are HIV-positive. I called the U.S. Military Entrance Processing Station (MEPS) in Baltimore, Maryland, and they told me that you cannot enter into the military when you are already HIV-positive.

When I joined the military, I was very apprehensive about divulging my sexuality. It was very hard for me at first until I met someone. He seemed nice enough and he made his move on me when we were at a party, upstairs watching TV. I did not know he was gay, but he was also in the military like me. We secretly started dating and then it became a violent situation, where he would threaten me and physically, emotionally, and mentally abuse me. He was in the military as well and so there was nowhere on base, I could hide from him. Eventually the situation alleviated itself and nobody in my command found out about it. If they had I would have been interrogated on our relationship and surely would have been kicked out. I had a bisexual girlfriend later on that year and we kept each other's secret until she was kicked out of the military because of "Don't Ask, Don't Tell." DADT was the policy that kept gays and lesbians from serving in the military openly. Since then, DADT has been eradicated and now one can serve openly as a gay man or lesbian.

Serving in silence is something that nobody should have to do. Right now, I serve under the Maryland Defense Force as a 1st Lieutenant, Communications Officer. The MDDF does not care if you are HIV-positive or gay—it is a volunteer service that serves to protect the borders of Maryland, alongside the National Guard and I am proud to serve openly and proudly as an HIV-positive gay man.

This entry of Just*in Time is dedicated to the men and women who serve or who have served our country, who are HIV-positive or HIV-negative.

Just*in Time: December 2012

December 24, 2012

by Justin B. Terry-Smith

**Dear Justin,**

**I have a question for you: What is your opinion about gift givers and bug chasers? I hear that there are people out there who want to spread HIV and others who are looking to get infected with HIV on purpose. I have been diagnosed with HIV for about one year now and I had to go on meds because I did not know I had it for so long. I hate taking them, but I know I have to in order to survive. I do not know anyone who would want to go through anything that I go through or anything you go through, either. I just do not get it. Can you give me some insight?**
**—Ali**

Let me first explain what a bug chaser is. A bug chaser is slang for someone who pursues sexual intercourse with people who are HIV-infected in order to eventually contract HIV. A gift giver is an HIV-positive person who wants to infect HIV-negative participants who willingly seek to become HIV-positive.

Well, when I first heard of bug chasers, I thought they were crazy. I really did not understand why someone would want to be infected with HIV. It is not until a close friend who is also HIV-positive talked to me about it that I understood more about it. He himself was a bug chaser at one point in time, until he was diagnosed with HIV himself.

Here is what might be one reason why people "chase" HIV. The HIV community has been through a lot since HIV/AIDS had been discovered and named. Some people who are negative view the community as one of acceptance, where one is able to be sexually free. Bug chasers, in my opinion, want to belong to a community and that need for belonging has somehow manifested itself as a need that is targeted towards the HIV community. Basically, some feel that being a part of the HIV community makes them a part of something special.

Another possible reason: Some bug chasers believe that getting HIV will make safe sex a moot point, and so, therefore, in this mentality, they believe that catching HIV is getting rid of any anxiety of always having to worry about catching HIV. Obviously, some of them have not contracted other viruses like hepatitis C, or they would realize that they are at risk for other infections like a different, possibly drug-resistant, strain of HIV. In my opinion, these men probably do not want HIV, but they think it will happen no matter what they do sexually.

Loneliness also may have something to do with it, as well. A lot of these men do not want to die alone or at least want to control their own destinies when it comes to death. Death comes for everyone, but with suicide, for example, a lot of people believe that at least death is on your own terms and nobody else's.

And in some countries being HIV-positive may put you in front of the line for some healthcare benefits and services.

Also, a lot of people feel that society has treated them like crap, and they feel liberated about being positive because they feel that HIV has shown them how to be stronger and to find themselves as well. When someone feels like they are a part of a society so strongly, it hurts when that society shuns them. For example, religion gives a lot of people a sense of who they are and a sense of belonging. When a person is shunned for their religion, they will try to look for something to fill that empty void; they will look to another community for that same sense of belonging.

All in all, when anyone is infected no matter how, it is a travesty. To have someone willing to infect another with "the gift" of HIV is just as awful. This is not a gift and, trust me, I think it sucks…Merry Christmas, Happy Kwanzaa, Happy Chanukah, and Happy New Year. But remember, some gifts are just not supposed to be opened.


Just*in Time: January 2013
January 23, 2013

Just*in Time by Justin B. Terry-Smith

**Good Evening Justin,**

**I said this before, but it just seems like I know you—it is your smile. But this is the reason for this message: I am living with HIV as are a couple of my friends. Now, one thinks that people who have sex without disclosing should be jailed and that people who are living with the virus who do not work should be put on an island in a federal homeless shelter instead of given housing. He believes this will stop the spread of HIV in the young Black MSM (men who have sex with men) community. He tells me to stop telling him it will not work and tell him what will and, honestly, I do not know. But I do know that dehumanizing and incarcerating is not the answer. Any suggestions?**

**—Ron**

Okay, first of all, let us get something straight. Your friend that is saying all these horrible things needs help. All these things are in his head, but did you ever think of why? There could be something there besides the reason of lowering HIV infection rates among the Black MSM community. He might be going through some self-loathing himself. But let us look at this on the other side of things as well.

So, why would someone actually say that people who do not disclose should be jailed and that people who are living with the virus who do not work should be put on an island in a federal homeless shelter instead of given housing?

(As an aside to this last suggestion, let me just say that there are people who take advantage of the system, but if your friend wants to put them on an island, he will have to put everyone that does not want to work on an island. I do not know anyone who really wants to go to work.)

There are always two sides to every argument and then the truth, and you have to figure that out yourself. As you might know I have been out with my HIV status since I was diagnosed in 2006. One of the only reasons why I was so comfortable about disclosing my HIV status is because I had friends who were HIV-positive since the age of nineteen and I even dated one of them. So, because I was exposed to people living with HIV, I did not feel funny about meeting or dating them. That being said since your friend is HIV-positive, I am going to guess he might not have had a lot of HIV-positive friends who are open and comfortable with their own status.

Okay, now, how he was infected really has to be considered. If he was betrayed by a boyfriend or someone, he dated that might make him bitter. As a lot of us know having your heart broken can really cut someone deep; now add that the person who broke your heart also infected you with HIV.

BURRRNNNNN!!! OUUCHHH!!! Cuts like a knife, doesn't it?

In my opinion I do not think jail and deportation is the answer to solve anyone's issues, especially not HIV within the Black MSM community. I am open about my status because I am comfortable, man; others are not. Why might others not be comfortable about disclosing their HIV status to their sexual partners?

Well, we can say that the mentality that your friend has is exactly why they do not open up. That kind of mentality that your friend has feeds stigma, and that very stigma is why people who have HIV are in denial that they even have HIV and sometimes will engage in sexual activities without telling anyone about their own HIV status.

After all, how can one care for other people if one does not care about oneself?

Just*in Time: February 2013
February 18, 2013

**Justin:**
**I just have to say, I love you! I am writing because my son was in a two-year relationship, but they broke up this past May. After that, my son was dating a few different guys. As a mom, I kept giving him the talk about being careful and wearing protection if he had sex. My son is very open with me, and he did tell me he was not always wearing protection. Since October I have been on him about getting tested because he was putting himself at risk.**

**On November 7, he got a call from the doctor telling him he was positive. I have been asking my son to go to the Web site, thebody.com, and watch your videos, but he will not have any part of that. He just keeps telling me he is fine. My son thinks he does not have HIV. He did have a Western blot done, so I know the test is not wrong.**

**I am just worried that my son will go into a depression soon. He will not go to any support groups and he does not want to talk about it unless he brings it up. My son has support from me, the family, and a few good friends that he did tell. I am worried about how he really is feeling inside, though. What can I do to help my son?**

**Also, my son wants to stay on dating sites and meet people. I am scared that he is just going to get hurt more. I know if he meets someone and he tells them he is positive they will not want to be with him. I did ask him to join an HIV dating site, but he says he does not think there are any and he does not want to date someone that is poz. Is that normal to think that way at first? And how can I get him to connect with other people who are going through the same thing he is?**

**Thank you for your time Justin and thank you for being there for so many others…you are an amazing person!**
**—Christine**

First let me just say that you are a good mother. I love that you felt open and trusting enough to send me this letter. My mother also was scared for me and gave me the talk about protected sex and being careful. But, as adults, we are in charge of making our own way and making our own decisions.

Finding out that you are positive may be jarring when you first hear it. One might go into denial or a state of numbness to where you will think nothing of it. Or even going as far as forgetting you even have the disease because the emotions of being scared, feared, and unloved are so impactful that one will say, "I'm fine," when you are really not.

He sounds like he is going through deep depression and is not snapping out of it anytime soon. He will have to let it out some way. I am most worried about that he will find another way, a more dangerous way, to let out his frustrations. In my life drugs and sex seemed to cover up a lot of pain and sorrow. He will need to find a way.

I would also check to see if he is suffering from low self-esteem. There are many poz dating sites on the Internet. Before I met my husband, I met a lot of guys off dating sites that did not care about my HIV status because they liked me for me. Depending on his age a lot of young people do like going through the Internet to connect to other people that are going through the same things they are.

Ask him why he would not want to date someone who is poz. It is a case-by-case basis about the feelings one has about being poz. There is no feeling that is normal or abnormal. You need to just be there and reassure him that you will always be there.

Just\*in Time: March 2013

March 29, 2013

**Justin:**

**I am HIV-positive; I was diagnosed April 2012. I think I have dealt with my diagnosis very well. But I do have my moments of weakness. Last night I was talking to a guy who is a good friend who I am in love with. We have been seeing each other since the summer of 2012. I stopped seeing him in September 2012 because once we both admitted our feelings he started to change. He began to distance himself. So, I just cut it off because if you do not want to be with me, I am not going to fight with you to change your mind. I have a life I have to live. And dreams I want to flourish.**

**After not talking for a few months, he asked me out on a date in December, where he told me that he loved me and that we had a connection he did not want to lose. So, I naturally was shocked and happy because he opened up and actually said that. So, I kind of have been playing it safe with him because I do not want to give my heart to him and get let down again. So last night I was speaking to him and I asked him two questions—how he feels about my status, because he has known from the very beginning; and how he feels after we have sex, because he and I have had sex a total of three times. And we have not used condoms. In the moment I do not think either of us thinks about it. But after, it weighs heavily on my heart because I love this boy and I would not wish this disease on my worst enemy, let alone someone I love.**

**So, he responded the way I assumed he would. We both agreed to use condoms. And he says the only time my status is a problem is when we have had unprotected sex. So, then**

our conversation ventured into another topic and he randomly says, "We can't have sex anymore. I cannot have sex for a while. I need to stop for like six months. So, I can stay focused on the things I need to do."

Naturally, it made me feel like he did not want me at all because of my status and now I am a little fucked up about it. And I am on my way back home to NYC and I do not want to be in this mode. Have you ever dealt with this or known someone who has? What did you or they do?
—Thomas

First, let me say I am happy that you seem at peace with your status as it is very hard even after a year of being diagnosed to be able to deal with it. But I think the reality that he did not use condoms while having sex with someone who is HIV-positive may have scared him a little bit. I noticed that there was nothing in your e-mail about getting tested for HIV. You need to make sure he is getting tested for HIV.

I understand that you do not want to wish this on anyone and neither do I. If he needs six months to think it over, give him his time, but not too much. For me, baby, I wait for no man and I do not think a man should wait for me. If he really loves you for you, despite your HIV, he will come back to you. If he does not come back to you, you will be fine. There will be another man out there for you that will not need a six-month break. You see, home is where the heart is, whether or not it has HIV in it. I would also advise that you occupy your time doing something you love…other than him! But seriously, he might be just a little freaked out now, so just relax and take your time.

Just*in Time: April 2013
April 24, 2013

Just*in Time
by Justin B. Terry-Smith

**Hi Justin,**

**I am struggling because I recently found out that my boyfriend tested positive for HIV during our relationship. It has been six months to date since this happened & I am still dealing with the situation mentally. When I first got the news, I was getting tested every two weeks and about two months ago I have limited it to once a month. All of my tests have been negative, but, for some reason, I am dealing with anxiety issues to the max. I feel like every symptom is there and I am having it. I do not understand why I cannot move on from this. Getting tested should be helping me but it just takes me back to the same place I was when I first got the news. Maybe you can give me some words of wisdom and encouragement that will help me to move past this & move on. Oh, and now I am terrified to have sex. I do not sleep around I was always in a relationship so I do not understand why me…so maybe you can help.**
**—Monique**

Let me start out by saying that you have to stay strong. It is very hard getting out of this stage. The not knowing can be very tough to get through, but you can get through this and you will get through this.

Whether or not the test ever comes back positive or remains negative, you will be okay. HIV most of the time will take longer than two months to show up in any blood test. I do not know what symptoms you might have but I am going to guess that you are questioning just about everything that might be happening to your body right now. The key is to stay calm, and do not worry until there is something to worry about.

Also, you must feel very betrayed right now—that I understand—but we must put attention where it would benefit everyone and that is on the virus. We need to blame the virus and not others. I suggest therapy as well because it does truly help you move forward. Yes, there might be a time period where you are afraid to have sex with anyone, but in time that might pass. A lot of people have the misconception that HIV only infects people who are promiscuous which is NOT the case. People in "monogamous" relationships can be infected with HIV as well. Stay strong, Monique, be calm and keep in mind this motto that has always helped me get through life: Worry about the things you have control over and do not worry about the things you do not. Be brave, baby. Hugs and kisses!

**Justin—**

**Justin, I think I could learn a lot from you. I seldom disclose my status to anyone, including a few that I have had "close encounters" with. I am in fear of doing so. Although, the few times that I have told my partners about it, they replied, "Don't worry, I have it to." Unfortunately, the disease affects more than we give it credit for....**

Back to me—I am afraid of being alienated by my family and friends. I have lived with this for twelve years now, so you think I would be comfortable with it. Anything that you have to share with me would be greatly appreciated. Thank you, Justin.
—Chad

I understand about only disclosing to those who you are intimate with. Fear is the ultimate enemy. In the 1980s–90s and even now people are afraid of losing their jobs, friends, family, and their very lives if they disclose their status. I have always been the kind of guy to stand up for what I believe in even if that means losing people I love. I would start small by telling someone who you know. The more you tell people the easier it gets. I am not saying, shout it from the rooftops, but maybe we should start with a whisper. When you throw the tiniest pebble in a pond, it makes ripples. But those ripples expand throughout the pond. If they have a problem with it remember it is those people who have the problem and not you. SMOOTCHIES

Just*in Time: May 2013

May 17, 2013

Just*in Time by Justin B. Terry-Smith

**Hello Justin,**

**I do admire you so much! I added you as a friend [on Facebook] but never wanted to patronize you by coming up with clichés.**

I am an African woman living in the U.K. I have a big family as you can imagine…and I have a cousin who I have supported since he lost his father at the age of eight years. I am turning forty this August and, for me, he is the son I was meant to have even though I am only eleven years older than him. I knew he was gay before he realized it himself. But I let him be so that he could find his own way.

From his first experience, he contracted HIV; now the challenge is saving him! I am doing my best—he is ok as he is on a therapy that is, for now, supporting his immune system! Unfortunately, in our family, there is no room for a gay man let alone one with HIV! I love my little because, and I will support him till the end of my life (I am constantly researching new discoveries!). I am here for him and I am glad you are here for everyone…keep being you and be the best you can be! But do not forget to live. Anything I could do to give him more support? —Hannah xoxo

Let me first say thank you so much for being so real with me in your approach. It is amazing to see someone who has taken this young man and stood in as one of his parents when he had none.

They say that usually mothers know about their child's sexuality even before the child does. My parents did the same with me. They knew I was gay but let me find my own way in my own sexuality.

I am very sorry that he contracted HIV, and I am glad you do not feel guilty about it. My parents, I know, felt guilty when they were informed, I was HIV-positive. I told them that they did nothing wrong and that they had nothing to do with my contracting HIV.

By therapy I think you mean treatment, and this is good. Remember, though, that he needs to stay on that treatment, and he might want to seek out a counselor or someone to talk to when he feels a little depressed.

Family can be tough at times. Remember to be there for him and make sure he knows that you are there for him. He might not want to talk about it now with you, but he will eventually come around. When my mother was told about my HIV status, I had not had a chance to tell her myself. It turns out my own cousin told her mother, who told my mother.

I got a phone call from my family with all of them crying on speaker phone. They asked me sobbing, "Do you have AIDS? We heard you had AIDS!"
I replied, "No I do not have AIDS."

They asked again, "Justin do you have HIV?"

Then I replied, "Yes I have HIV."

They started crying even more.

I told them, "You have to be strong with me and not cry for me."

After that moment they stopped crying and started supporting. For example, my mother and other family members sponsor me for the Washington, D.C. AIDS Walk/5K. They call to check up on me and they still treat me the same as if I did not have HIV.

For more support I would suggest that he find a support group. Depending on age/race, etc., he might feel more comfortable with a certain demographic. The analogy that I made up is "Being with others in the same boat might make you want to paddle faster to get to your destination." It might help him stick to his treatment regimen and keep his doctor's appointments, as well.

It sounds like you love him like a mother would and I think that is fantastic. Happy Mother's Day!

Just*in Time: June 2013
June 12, 2013

Jus*in Time by Justin B. Terry-Smith

**Justin—**
**I am twenty-seven years young. I contracted HIV on February 15, 2010, from a guy who did not tell me but then maybe I really did not want to know. As a child, I had neither self-**

confidence nor self-esteem. My parents moved me from school-to-school thinking that that would help the problem. I was a gay man and not the most masculine of men, but I was in a phase of trying to find out who I was and trying to fit in, which never worked.

It got worse. It got harder as I got older. Until last year, I did not like much about myself. I was not trying at all. Becoming HIV-positive helped to change my attitude somewhat because it gave me a different lease on life. My mother says it humbled me completely.

My mother and I talk, and she asks questions and makes sure I am doing all I can to help myself. My father is different now. We have a better relationship now after HIV than I had before. Now I am on a kind of journey, searching for my sense of self all over again.

I met a guy. He is ten years older and a nice guy. Well, we have been sexual for over three years off and on. He was not the one who gave me HIV. He does not know. I have pushed people away trying to not be in a relationship. I never thought I was ready. I always ask people about relationships and love....What's it like to love someone or be in love? For the first time ever, I could see myself happy with him. I do not know if I should tell him the truth. I am afraid he will walk away for good. I do not know what to do. I am so scared because I think I am in love, but I do not know if it is an infatuation or hormones or HIV. He may be the only man who sees me for me. I do not want to lose that part. This is really the first time we are communicating and that is why I wonder more [about a possible future].

On your blog, I listened to how you met your husband. I wonder if that is possible for me.
—Dimitri

The funny thing about disclosure is that you are damned if you do and damned if you do not.

Okay, let us break this, down shall we? Be very careful about what you are doing. In some states it is illegal not to disclose your HIV status to your sexual partners. People have gone to jail on even just a rumor of them not disclosing their status to their sexual partner. Also, make sure you consider that he might be okay with you being HIV-positive but not okay with you not being upfront with him. There is also the factor that he might be mad at you for not disclosing. You will never know unless you are able to tell him about your status.

I suggest telling him in a very safe environment. Take it upon yourself to educate him if he is not educated. Be prepared for both positive and negative responses. LOVE is possible though you should have enough esteem in yourself to walk away in case this does not work out.

There is someone out there for everyone. Sometimes it takes a little longer to find them. You are a very young man, and you have a lot of time for love. I met my husband around your age, and I told my husband about my status the first night I met him, and he still wanted me.

Trust me, you will find that dream man you want—just take your time. Older men tend to have a better understanding of HIV, because they have been around to see the transition of different perceptions of HIV. If you think you are in love, love him enough to tell him the truth. Lastly, the more confidence and self-esteem you have the more comfortable you yourself will be with your own disclosure.


Just*in Time: July 2013

July 13, 2013

Just*in Time by Justin B. Terry-Smith

**Justin—**
**We actually know each other on Facebook and throughout the community, but I wanted to write you this letter in confidence.**

**My partner and I moved away to work on our relationship and now we are considering moving back to the area. After many discussions, my partner is finally opening up to the idea of polyamory. I have been a polyamorist for a long time and my partner did not like the idea of a third person in our relationship, but now, since we have talked, he is open to the idea.**

**Well, we have found a third, but there is a slight problem. He likes to bareback. Since we are all trying to keep each other HIV-negative, my boyfriend and I refuse to have unprotected sex with him.**

**Let me say, he agreed that he will not have unprotected sex with me or my boyfriend because he does not want to hurt us in any way. He is HIV-negative and only has bareback sex with guys who tell him that they are undetectable, and he gets tested every six months. I understand that may lower the risk of HIV transmission, but I am still feeling kind of funny about it.**

**What should I do? Any advice is greatly appreciated.**

**—PC**

As a polyamorist myself, I feel first we need to describe what polyamory is to our readers. Polyamory is the practice, desire, or acceptance of having more than one intimate relationship at a time with the knowledge and consent of everyone involved. Okay, so are we all on the same page? Great!! Now back to you, Mac—I mean, PC.

The fact that you and your partner are agreeing to this makes me feel happy because it means that the lines of communication are open. A lot of couples go through this and suffer permanent damage from either party not being able to convey the kind of love they want.

Okay, he is having unprotected sex with guys who tell him they are undetectable. So, you know they could be lying just to have sex, right? I would advise him of that and make sure he gets tested every three months and not six months; to me, early detection of any health issue is key to survival.

I suggest having a sit-down talk with him, your boyfriend, and yourself. This will give you the opportunity to talk things through with all parties represented. Communicate your fears and concerns with the issue; after all, HIV is not the only STI you would have to worry about. Now, if you can deal with him having unprotected sex outside of your relationship, okay, but, if you are still feeling funny about it, then there could be a molehill that could have the potential to be a mountain of a problem. Remember: Polyamory is a serious relationship among individuals who must honor each other with perfect love and perfect trust.

My husband and I are polyamorist and protect each other and other people. We have been open and honest with each other from the very beginning about what and who we want. There are others (who shall remain nameless) who are not as honest, but we are always continuing to explore different avenues of love. Judging others because they are getting the love, they want will not get us anywhere. Having an open dialogue will let us learn and teach us how to protect ourselves from HIV and other STDs, no matter what kind of relationship we are in.

Being polyamorist does not spread HIV. Having an honest relationship will allow that polyamorist relationship to remain strong and defend itself against STI/STDs—but only if all parties are honest. We need that strength because we still live in a society that looks down upon polyamory in some respects. Let me know what happens!


Just*in Time: August 2013
August 8, 2013

Just*in Time
by Justin B. Terry-Smith

**Justin,**

**I am sure you get lots of messages but wanted to say thanks for your videos and really good support they have given me. Every little bit helps. People like you are so needed. I got into the "system" by a surprise HIV diagnosis a month ago; it has been tougher than I thought but I am stronger than I expected so it is okay.**

**You are one of three people who have put really good things on-line. It is strange almost because through work I come across stories about HIV and things all the time. I work in the Web hosting department for a U.S. TV/media company so I will hopefully be over in**

the U.S. soon, and, actually, I have a "brother" (from another mother) in L.A., where I go a lot. I love how the U.S. has changed attitudes and hope to be there for good one day. London is okay but getting too crowded and, being Swedish, I miss nature and the ocean.

I do have just a quick question; maybe there is no easy answer. Suppose one meets a guy and everything goes really well but you need to tell him about the little blue devils (you know what I mean). Ugh, I should have said it upfront. One of my mates said, "You tell and if he doesn't understand then he won't be right anyway."
—Jonas
London, United Kingdom

Your friend is right. I think the proper thing to do in these matters is to disclose, especially if you have already been intimate. But why not disclose before you are intimate so that he knows what he is getting himself into? Not saying that having a partner who is HIV-positive is an issue, but to start off open and honest about your status is, in my opinion, the right thing to do.

There is also a time and place to do everything. I suggest that you may want to feel around the question about HIV and see if he is okay with it by either coming straight out and telling him or being very cautious. There are many different ways to tell someone but be careful, especially if you have already been intimate. I do not know what the laws are in the U.K. but we here in the United States have what we call HIV criminalization laws. These laws persecute anyone who does not tell their sexual partners that they themselves are HIV-positive.

If he does not understand that, then do not worry about it; I know there are plenty of men in the sea (or the English Channel) for you. Also make sure you take care of yourself and go to the doctor. A new HIV-positive diagnosis can make people feel like HIV is something they can write off. Take care of yourself first. You cannot take care of anyone unless you take care of yourself first.

[UPDATE]

Hey Jonas,

How is it going with the HIV diagnosis and did my advice help?

—Justin

**Justin,**

**People get complacent with HIV and they think it is no big deal but, in my case, it caused early inflammation of the brain. I have had terrible headaches for the past months and they finally put me on meds now and hopefully they will improve. I nearly panicked at the waiting room for the meds, realizing this is really happening, and, when I took them for the first time, it really, really sunk in because in the back of my head there was always a slight denial that maybe I did not have it. Now I feel great relief; this thing is being taken care of and I can live my life again.**

**Now about the boyfriend: I told him, and he is fine and wants to marry me. Thank you for asking me it means a lot. The only problem is I was going to leave London—now I am rethinking all of it. I know it is silly giving up my dreams of L.A. for a man, but I think he is worth it.**

**—Jonas**

Just*in Time: September 2013

September 6, 2013

**Just*in Time**

by Justin B. Terry-Smith

**Justin,**

**Hello, I have tried to send you a friend request after I sent this message because I thought I would ask you for permission to become your friend on Facebook. I really admire you as far as the work that you do for the HIV and gay community.**

**I just wanted to share with you that I am a very closet-type person. I do not know a lot of people, strictly by choice. I am gay—not DL (down low) or bisexual, but gay. Because of the**

**lack of education that people have and their stupidity about it, I keep it to myself. July 22nd will make ten years for me being HIV-positive. Never have had to take medication, never have been hospitalized for it and that is a blessing.**

**I have a personal issue about something, and I know I can get an honest answer from you. Why is Magic Johnson the face of HIV or whenever they use somebody it is always like that? Let me explain. Why does the media or news outlets never show the truth about HIV, you know, the having to take pills, and the going to the clinic, and being hospitalized? Why is the hardcore stuff never shown? Personally, I think it would help if it were really shown how HIV breaks your body down. Well, thank you for your time. I really appreciate all that you do you.**
**—DD**

First let me say thank you so much for e-mailing me. Facebook will only allow a certain number of friends per person (hint, hint: try looking up J.B. Terry-Smith).

Well, I can see you have a loaded question that could have a lot of different answers. You have to take into consideration that Magic Johnson was one of the first professional athletes to come out and say that he was infected with the virus. In 1991 that was almost unheard of and it took a lot of bravery and courage to openly tell the public about his HIV status, especially being a celebrity and professional athlete. I believe he helped a lot of people in encouraging them to disclose their status or get tested or go for treatment.

Johnson retired in the same year but came back to play in an All-Stars game in 1992. Now, twenty-two years after his HIV disclosure he has given his time and energy into raising money for HIV/AIDS awareness. Also let me say to my other readers that just because he is still living does not mean in any way, shape, or form he is free of HIV or cured. It just means he has taken care of himself and also has the money to do so.

It is now 2013 and he is no longer "the face of HIV" in my opinion; anyone who is open with their status, not only to their partners, friends, and family but to the world, is "a face of HIV." There is no one specific person who could hold that title. That being said, celebrities and athletes are able to raise awareness of a disease a lot faster than people in the general population. People in the general population usually listen to people like Magic Johnson, Ellen, Don Lemon, Anderson Cooper, etc., because they are trusted spokespersons on issues that affect us all. Over time media outlets have shown people infected with HIV in the hospital, taking HIV medications, etc., but now we have YouTube where we ourselves can show the truth about HIV. I know on my YouTube channel I show all of those things. But that is only my truth about HIV, there are several others like myself, Robert Breining, Patrick Rio Kay, Mark S. King, Marvelyn Brown, Maria Mejia, Dab Garner, Jose Ramirez, Anthony Polimeni, Aaron Laxton, AJ King, etc., who are faces of HIV activism. We do not have the money other (famous) spokespeople might have, or get the recognition we deserve, but our hearts are just as big if not bigger. We are all dedicated to eradicating this disease from our communities and from the earth.

Now, my question to you, DD, and to the rest of my readers is: What are you doing to help fight HIV in your community?

Keep on fighting the good fight and we will win the war.

Just*in Time: October 2013
October 18, 2013

**Just*in Time**
by Justin B. Terry-Smith

**Justin,**
**I was recently diagnosed with HIV and I have been dealing with it pretty well but there are still times—at least once or twice a day—when I feel insecure or down about the situation. I have basically come to terms with the fact that I have HIV and the fact that I made a mistake. I have been looking for validation that I can live a long life with medication and taking care of myself. I read so many things on-line looking for answers, some of them encouraging and making sense and some that speak gloom and doom and make me feel like, even though I am taking medicine, AIDS is coming, and my time is short. I refuse to listen to anything that speaks that kind of negativity, but it is not always that easy being strong, considering this is still new and I have really no one to talk to or relate to about this.**

**Another thing, Justin, is that I am afraid I will never find a soul mate. I felt inspired watching your videos on YouTube and discovering that you have a husband, but I feel like it was hard finding a guy that acts right without HIV in the picture let alone when it is (LOL). It really gets to me sometimes. I know you are busy and have a lot going on yourself, but if you find time soon to respond you will hopefully let me know how silly I am being (LOL). I would appreciate it and thank you for everything you are doing to encourage those dealing with this and for being so brave.**

**God bless you—hope to hear from you soon.**

**Sincerely, James**

You are not being silly. I honestly think you are doing the right thing. I think that taking out the negativity in your life is a very important thing, not only because you are living with HIV, but because you are living.

I have had to cut close friends out of my life because of the negativity they brought or bring into my life and I will continue to do so. It is very important that HIV-infected people do this, because a big part of being infected with HIV is mental. Keeping positive about living can affect how your body will deal with HIV and other infections.

Taking your HIV medications is a big part of the physical part of it. Continue to take your medications! Trust me, I have a lot of friends who denied they had HIV and refused medication even after their positive diagnosis. They have since passed and some continue to die. I think of Josh, Leon, Rodney, Patrick, and many others who didn't even make it to their twenties, so heed my warning and take your meds.

As for love, that is a different conversation, so let us talk about it, shall we? Okay, this is a big concern to a lot of HIV-positive people. In my opinion I would always try to be open in the beginning, because if they have an issue with me being positive then I am glad I found out in the beginning, so I do not waste my time; if all they see is HIV when they look at me then what is the point of even going on a second date? You will find your soul mate—just keep that positivity going.

**Justin:**

**I am doing great. Thank you so much for getting back to me and following up to see if I am**

okay. I was going through a bit of a culture shock when I found out, but I am healthy and loving life. I do struggle with trying to date and find someone and also feel a little insecure about talking about my status with anyone because people judge. Any suggestions?
James

My suggestion is: "Fuck 'em!" Anyone who is going to judge you because you have HIV can kiss my black, gay, author, activist, married, parenting HIV-positive ass. You will always have HIV (unless there is a cure) whether or not you decide to speak openly about it with anyone. The choice is ultimately yours, but the more you speak openly about it, the more comfortable you will be.

Just*in Time: November 2013

November 25, 2013

**Just*in Time**

by Justin B. Terry-Smith

**Hey Justin,**

**How are you? I really enjoy your videos and I admire your strength.**

**My issue is that I am a twenty-one-year-old transgender female, and I am scared I may be positive. A couple months ago I got bumps on my left breast that turned into a scab; I scrubbed the scab off, and my skin never healed. A couple days ago I had smaller bumps pop up (one turned into a scab) and the others are very tiny sores; I went to the urgent care clinic in my area and they did not even know what it really was. They labeled it dermatitis, so I let it go and, later, decided to get an HIV test. I was talking to my friend who was a nursing student, and he said this condition normally occurs in people with HIV (I did not tell him it was me, though).**

**I am scared because if I am positive, then this is not something that I want anybody to know. I want it to be a secret until the day I die. I am used to being the pretty girl and**

**getting a lot of compliments and attention and I know a lot of people would feel as though I deserved it or would not look at me the same anymore. I cannot tell my mother or father as they are very uneducated about HIV—they think you can get HIV from sharing a pizza with a person who has it, so imagine how they would treat me? I had a former friend who has HIV, but we no longer speak, and I do not know if I could trust him with this because he is very open about his own status.**

**I know you are a very busy person but, please, if you are ever on-line, can you check on me every once in a while? You are the only person I can talk to.**

**—TG Sexy**

I am doing fine, but it sounds like you need some advice. We will have to address one problem at a time.

Dermatitis is not caused by HIV. Dermatitis is simply inflammation of the skin; there are many things that can cause dermatitis. Some metals, fiberglass, rubber, perfumes, etc., can cause the inflammation. I know for a fact that I love wearing silver, but it is silver-plated material that makes me break out. Every time I wore a silver-plated chain around my neck, I needed cream prescribed by a doctor. Dermatitis can also be caused by outside irritants like bleach, soaps, detergents, and other cleaning supplies. It also can be caused by stress or a vitamin deficiency. Go see your doctor to get properly diagnosed and treated for dermatitis.

I know you are scared, but my motto is: Only worry about something when there is something to worry about. You must get tested. Now, I know that is hard to do but you must do it. If it is negative, you will be okay. If the test is positive, then the earlier you know, the better. The more time that goes by that you are untreated for HIV, the more you open yourself up to infections and other complications from the virus.

It sounds like people around you are ignorant about HIV. I suggest if you are HIV-positive you may want to find a group of people that is supportive because you will need them in your network. Be careful about whom you confide in, but you must find support in groups of like-minded people.

Again, if the test is positive, you might want to look at it as another chance at life. Think about the different ways HIV will make you focus on your health and happiness. You will find solace as long as you focus on the positive things you get from this very experience. Life does not stop because you have HIV; you have to live on for you and all the transgender men and women out there who are HIV-positive. Be an example of a healthy, HIV-positive beautiful girl that you know, and I know you are, inside and outside.

You are a wonderful transgender woman and fuck all the haters. Get up and get tested. Love you!


Just*in Time: December 2013
December 27, 2013

**Hey Justin,**
**I was date raped and I had experienced what is called oral thrush. I got tested for HIV when I had thrush and the test came out negative. I think it is a rare strain of thrush. I cannot get diagnosed with HIV, and I am very depressed and do not know how often to check my immune system for HIV. I just want closure.**
**—Conrad**


First things first, I am very sorry about what happened to you. Let me just say that I can empathize with you when it comes to the subject of rape. I have my own experience with rape and the first thing I recommend is to get past the fact that it actually happened, and it is not your fault. I do not know the details of the crime that happened to you, but it is a start.

Now for some of our readers who do not know what thrush is, let me explain. According to the CDC, thrush, or oropharyngeal/esophageal candidiasis is a type of fungus that lives in the mouth/throat/tongue. It looks like white patches, almost like the canker sores that you get throughout your mouth. Thrush usually does not happen in healthy adults. Individuals that are diagnosed with thrush usually have associated health issues, such as HIV/AIDS, cancer treatments, organ transplantation, diabetes, corticosteroid use, dentures and/or broad-spectrum antibiotic use. To prevent thrush, you must maintain good oral hygiene and use mouthwash.

Now, Conrad, back to you. Before I was HIV-positive, I got tested every three months. Even though you are scared of getting tested and being HIV-positive you need to know. The earlier you know, the better you can take care of yourself. Whether the diagnosis is positive or negative you need to know. If you go through life running from everything you are scared of, you will be running for the rest of your life. The first step is to get tested, and then figure out whether you have something to worry about. And, hey, if it is a positive HIV test you still might not have anything to worry about. Just live life to the fullest. Thank you so much for writing in—I hope this helps.

**Justin,**

**Hi, there. I finally got to watch your "Who infected me with HIV?" video and I was wondering if there is a way to test for which strain you have and compare it to the two guys, one of whom may have infected you? Or does HIV mutate too much to do that? Just a thought, I hope you are doing well! Muah!**
**—Gina B.**

Let me explain to some of my readers what Gina means by the "Who infected me with HIV?" video. Recently I found out that the person, whom I had thought infected me with HIV, may have not been the person who infected me with HIV. Someone with whom I had sexual intercourse at that same time reminded me of a sexual encounter we had with each other where no condom was used. In response to this discovery, I had to share my feelings. I did a video on YouTube in response to my feelings, entitled "Justin's HIV Journal: Who infected me with HIV?" to share my thoughts about this particular subject matter.

There is no test to tell you when you were infected with HIV. I have researched this and have yet to find any such test. But there is a way to find out which strain of HIV you have. The test that you might be thinking of is called the genotype test for HIV. This should be administered to everyone who tests positive for HIV. The reason why is because this test will tell the doctor and patient what medication they might need to be on. For example, some HIV strains are resistant to some HIV medications. Doctors will have to look at the genotype test of the HIV-positive patient to determine which HIV medications will work with that strain of HIV. Not all HIV medications will work with all strains of the virus. I hope I was able to answer your question. I am doing well, along with my husband and son. Thank you for asking. XOXOX

Just*in Time: January 2014

January 25, 2014

**Hello Justin,**

**My name is Enrique and I live in Mexico and I am HIV-positive. I first saw your blog and YouTube videos around two years ago, or maybe more. That is when I first got diagnosed and I started looking things up on the Internet and I was led to your YouTube blog. Well, I have a question for you if you do not mind me asking.**

**I am currently on [a combination of antiretrovirals], and all has been okay until recently my kidneys have been pulsing, though pretty mildly. I am already trying to change a lot of things for that and I will consult my doctor to see if they need to change my meds.**

**What I really wanted to ask you concerns my family. I have two daughters in the United States of America. They are seventeen and sixteen; they are American citizens and so is my sister. My mom and brother also live in San Antonio, Texas. I am waiting to see if immigration reform gets passed this year, and, if it does, there is a high chance that I may be able to go home. If not, then I will be forced to cross the border illegally to get back with my family. I have been away from them for ten years and I cannot take it anymore. I am at the point of having suicidal thoughts and being depressed, but I am still hanging in there.**

**Now to my question: If I were to cross illegally or even legally, what are my options to get HIV meds at no cost or low cost. Like, let us say I was completely illegal; is there any nonprofit agency that would help me get meds? That is one of my main concerns.**

**Well, I hope you are doing well friend and I hope to hear back from you…god bless.**

**—Enrique**

Hola, Enrique. ¿Cómo estás? First, let me say thank you so much for reaching out to me. I have never been to Mexico and I had to do some research before responding. Let me just do an intro to our readers first.

According to the AIDS Healthcare Foundation (AHF), about 0.3 percent of adults in Mexico are HIV-positive. Although that percentile is considered low, it has not decreased in over a decade.

According to UNAIDS (2010), Mexico stats are as follows:

• Population: 110.6 million
• People living with HIV: 220,000
• People receiving ARTs: 64,500

Even though 0.3 percent of adults in Mexico is considered a low number, HIV rates in rural areas continue to climb. According to a July 17, 2007 New York Times article, "Mexican Migrants Carry H.I.V. Home," one of the main causes for the rise of HIV in rural areas of Mexico are migrant workers. A lot of migrant workers from Mexico come into the United States for a long period of time. The reason why this happens is because migrant workers can earn more money working in the United States rather than strictly in Mexico; that way they can earn more money for their families. When the migrant workers are in the United States for a long period of time, they sometimes become infected with HIV; then, when the migrant workers go back to Mexico, they are bringing HIV back to their homes.

Now, Enrique, I am not saying or asking how you contracted HIV; the most important thing is that you are receiving treatment. I am very glad that you are seeing a doctor about your issues with your kidneys; you might want to consider drinking more water as well. I remember when my doctor saw my kidney report and he suggested that I drink more and more water; it really helped my kidney functions.

Enrique, listen, I cannot legally tell you to cross the border or not to cross the border. But I can tell you this—your suicidal thoughts need to be addressed. I know that you have mentioned that you are seeking help physically, but you need to seek help mentally as well.

When you get to the United States, I would look into the Affordable Health Care Act, also known as Obamacare. Here is a Web site that can further assist you: www.healthcare.gov. To all my readers, whether you are insured or uninsured, illegal, or legal: Nobody should suffer while living with HIV/AIDS.

Just*in Time: February 2014

February 21, 2014

**Hello Justin,**

**Just checked out your video regarding the biohazard tattoo and it inspired me to write. I was diagnosed with HIV two years ago. When this happened, I did the responsible thing and notified those I had sexual relations with to ensure all were tested. I never was able to pinpoint who passed it to me but, to be honest, it does not matter. I accepted the issue and moved on accordingly. I often think about getting a biohazard tattoo myself because I do have multiple sex partners from time to time. I do practice safe sex.**

**I am in a fourteen-year open relationship with my wonderful partner. He knows my status and accepts it. However, from time to time, he insists on having unprotected sex. I am freaking out over this….I cannot bear the thought of passing this infection on to someone, let alone someone I love so much. For the time being I have convinced him to practice safe sex. Do you have any advice that can help when this issue comes up again?**

**I apologize in advance if the question is one you are uncomfortable answering, but I find myself alone when dealing with issues like this.**

**Need a little kind advice.**

**Thanks.**
**—J**

Let me say, fourteen years in a relationship is a very long time in "gay" years; you are like on your fiftieth anniversary…no, just kidding. CONGRATS!

Okay, let me first explain to my readers why I had a biohazard symbol tattooed on my abdomen. The reason why I had this done is because of what it meant to the gay community in the past and not what it means to many of us in the gay community now. I made a conscious decision to get the tattoo because it symbolized that I had HIV. A red ribbon is about HIV awareness and, yes, I could have gotten that, but I am not that kind of person.

In September 2013, I went through a spiritual awakening, so I had my biohazard covered with a Triquetra. A Triquetra represents the connection of mind, body, and soul, and in Celtic-based Pagan groups it is symbolic of the three realms of earth, sea, and sky. I also have the modern elemental symbols of Earth (Capricorn), my Sun Sign; Fire (Aries), my Rising Sign; and Fire (Aries), my Moon Sign. So, then I got a biohazard on my back because I still wanted it on my body but so that every time, I look in the mirror I will see spiritual inspiration. Some in the gay community use the biohazard symbol to mean that they bareback. I admit I have barebacked before but now I only bareback with my husband; I am no angel and I have made mistakes in the past.

In terms of using prevention tools, let me say that people are going to do what they want to do. Once you have voiced your opinion, that is about all you can or need to do. But you need to protect yourself. If this man loves you, he will not want to put your health in danger. I suggest getting tested for STIs more often. Honestly if he is doing it without you knowing there is a big trust and communication issue you might want to bring up. We who are HIV-positive are more susceptible to other STIs as well. If he is barebacking with others you really need to start taking precautions and talk to him about what he might be doing with others. If he says he wants to bareback with you, there should be something inside of you that asks, "WHY?" Also be informed that Truvada, as PrEP, is a drug that is used to protect people from getting infected with HIV but know that it is not indicated for protection against other STIs as well.

There are several types of viral hepatitis, such as A, B, C, D, E, G; the most common types are A, B, and C. The hepatitis viruses primarily attack the liver. Most of the individuals who are infected with hepatitis recover with a continuing immunity to the disease, but some people infected with the hepatitis virus die in the critical phase. Hepatitis B and C may develop to chronic hepatitis, in which the liver remains inflamed for more than six months. This can lead to cirrhosis, liver cancer, and sometimes death.

Also think about syphilis, drug resistant HIV, herpes, and chlamydia—which is not called the "Silent Killer" for nothing. THINK ABOUT IT!


Just*in Time: March 2014

March 1, 2014

**Hello Justin,**

**I have seen your Web site and it looks like you are a knowledgeable person about HIV and HIV prevention. I had a possible exposure with another male; I was the bottom partner and condoms were used, but it was my first experience, so I immediately got scared. Anyway, I went and got tested and was negative at three weeks and again at six weeks with a fourth-generation HIV test, which is conclusive at six weeks according to the clinic I went to. But just to be safe I tested at twelve weeks with the OraQuick oral swab and used your video to guide me and the result was negative again. So, do you believe that I should test again?**

**—Miguel**


Let us not go overboard here! I do believe in getting tested every three to six months.

There are several questions that you might ask after your potential exposure. How do you think you were exposed? When people talk about exposure, a lot of times they are thinking about unprotected sex. Some people think it means having sex with a condom. I bring this up because you cannot assess risk unless this question is answered, and it is not clear from your letter.

I see that you did use condoms, which is very effective when protecting yourself against HIV and other STIs (sexually transmitted infections). You are probably fine. You did a very good thing in being proactive when getting tested for HIV. You have consulted your clinic and they advised you correctly.

I understand the stress of having sex for the first time and the stress if you were exposed to HIV. But let us think calmly and rationally about this. It was your first time. Things are confusing right now, and you are scared, but it will pass with time. We have all had scares like this and nobody is immune to fearing the unknown. But the best advice I can tell you that was given to me is: "Why stress about something you can't do anything about?" My husband is the one who taught me that. Meaning, do not stress yourself out about whether or not you are positive or negative. Keep living your life and get tested every 3 to 6 months. According to the San Francisco AIDS Foundation:

"Antibody tests give a positive result based on antibodies to HIV, not the virus itself. 2-8 weeks (up to 2 months) after infection, most people will have enough antibodies to test positive. 12 weeks (3 months) after infection, about 97% of people will have enough antibodies to test positive.

"Antigen tests show a positive result based on the presence of the virus. These tests are more expensive than antibody tests, so are not offered in as many places. 1-3 weeks after infection, there will be enough viral material for a positive result.

"Polymerase chain reaction tests also test for the actual virus. This type of test is often used for testing the viral load of HIV-positive people, as well as testing babies born to HIV-positive mothers. 2-3 weeks after infection, there will be enough viral material for a positive result."

**Justin,**
**I was just wondering: Did your HIV provide additional problems when adopting a child? Just curious because this is something I wish to do.**
**—Prince**

Good question! Being HIV-positive, I did not think I would become a biological father at all. So, adoption was my option. I also did have the option of sperm cleansing and then going through an agency to find a surrogate to carry my child, but that costs thousands of dollars—so it was not a true option for me. My husband and I decided on adoption. On January 30, we adopted our son, Lundyn, who is a seventeen-year-old LGBT ball of hormones.

But to answer your question: No; I thought that having HIV would be an issue, but it was not. My husband and I went through the state of Maryland for our adoption. (Going through an agency would also cost money, but the state gives more benefits as far as education, food, and clothing allowances, etc., for the child.) The only thing they checked for when it came to my HIV infection was to make sure I was undetectable. I believe that the state wants to make sure that my HIV is under control and being undetectable proves to them that I am living healthy with HIV.

Just*in Time: April 2014

April 1, 2014

**Just*in Time**

by Justin B. Terry-Smith

**Hello Justin,**

**My condom broke and now I do not know what to do. What should I do? I am straight and I was having sex with my girl in her ass and it broke. I did not think I had any lube, so this time I just spit on the condom and used my saliva as lube. When I penetrated her, I did not really feel anything went wrong. After about an hour of having sex I ejaculated. But I did not know the condom had broken until after I pulled out of her. I then quickly ran to the bathroom and checked more thoroughly—and yes it broke indeed. I flushed the condom before my girlfriend saw me and I do not think she saw the condom after I pulled out of her.**

**I am very scared at this point. I hear that anal sex causes AIDS. Is that true? If it is, which one of us has it?**
**—Andre**

Okay, Andre, do not panic. As a member of the booty love fan club myself, I must say that I commend you on having the courage to write me. Not many straight guys do write in about the booty love, aka anal sex. Let me just say this, as a gay man I can say I have experience with the booty love.

Now, first things first. I believe you say in your e-mail, "I didn't think I had any lube, so this time I just spit on the condom and used my saliva as lube." I am guessing that this is not the first time you and your girlfriend have had anal sex, and you have used lube in the past. Lube has components that saliva does not, so, while saliva is very hot to use when having spontaneous sex, or even planned sex, it dries up a lot faster than lube does. In other words, using saliva means there is a greater chance that the condom will break.

Reconsider using lube when using a condom. There are tons of new lubes that are out now that anyone who lives in the United States with cable can see commercials for. They are also available at almost any drugstore. I suggest using AstroGlide or a product called Gun Oil—I know I like it. Wink!

And, dude, in my opinion you should tell your girlfriend what happened. That is my second suggestion. I know that you might be thinking that just because you cannot get her pregnant through anal sex, means it makes little difference if the condom broke or stayed intact. You are right about that one, my friend, but why would you try to hide the fact that the condom broke from her? It is okay to be honest with her. If she truly loves you, she will understand. I think you both should sit down and have a deep discussion about anal sex and then start exploring different types of lubrications and make it fun for her. This way you will not think you have to hide things from her.

The communication should always be open when it comes to sex with your partner(s). If you are not open about the love and sex you want from your partner(s) then you will not get the love or sex that you want. That might leave you a little high and dry…no pun intended…okay pun intended.

Okay, and, finally, anal sex itself does not cause AIDS. If you or your girlfriend do not have HIV than neither one of you can get HIV from each other. HIV is transmitted only if you are exposed to someone who already is infected with HIV. My suggestion is to get tested and make sure your girlfriend gets tested as well. Also, consider picking up some pamphlets about HIV transmission from the place where you usually get tested for HIV. If you do not have a place to get tested, you need to find one by going to A&U's locator or someplace similar on the Internet to search for it. It is best to know if you are HIV-positive or negative than to go on with life not knowing at all.

So, next time, remember: Lube it up before you beat it up!

For more information log on to the Centers for Disease Control and Prevention (CDC) Web site: www.cdc.gov/sexualhealth.

Just*in Time: May 2012
May 22, 2014

by Justin B. Terry-Smith

**Dear Justin,**
**I just found you on YouTube; I have been researching HIV a lot these past two weeks because my boyfriend just tested positive. I am scared shitless. I do not know what to do. We have been together for almost half a year now and have always used protection. I got tested last week and it was negative. My doctor thinks I am clean because it has been about six weeks since I last saw him. I have a follow-up next month, but now I am faced with a decision: What do I do now? I do not know how to navigate through this situation. I feel like I need to leave him, but I do not know how to get out because he keeps saying that I am only leaving because of his status. I am just scared. I have so many questions for you. If you have time, please hit me back. I feel helpless and lost.**

**—Gordon**

First, let me say: Breathe. Everything is going to be okay. Your partner is going to need someone to talk to and you might be the one that he needs. Make sure that you are there for support of him because he is going to need it. He needs to know that you are there for him and that this is not the end of the world.

Also, to make sure that you are okay, I would get tested again three months after the last HIV test you had. Also, let me say one thing about your doctor: I do not agree with the statement, "My doctor thinks I am clean because it has been about six weeks since I last saw him." HIV is a very tricky disease. You have to get tested again because HIV can be present in the body, sometimes without being detected. The window period (the time you need to wait to get an accurate test) for HIV is generally three months. I would recommend testing again at six months if the contact were very risky.

Whether or not you stay in this relationship is up to you. You need to make a choice whether you believe he is worth staying in this relationship for. My question would be: Has he broken your trust? If yes, it is going to be hard getting it back and do not let him claim that you are leaving him because of the HIV diagnosis—you would be leaving because he broke your trust, and, more importantly, your heart.

**Justin,**

**I am having a hard time. I was recently hospitalized with meningitis for eight days. There, they discovered that I had herpes. I am having such a hard time with this. It has been almost two months now. I am so upset with myself. The doctor said it was a new infection since I tested negative four weeks before. But my current partner tested negative. So, I am guessing it is from my ex…but he does not want to get tested for it. My doctor gave me pills for herpes, but says I only have to take them when I have an outbreak and he also told me the cream is ineffective. Tell me what to do?**

**—Matthew**

Ouchhh, meningitis! Well, let me say if the doctors did not tell you already that your herpes infection probably went untreated and that is probably why you have meningitis. I will say that being diagnosed with herpes is hard, but it is something that is manageable. Do not be upset with yourself because it will only feed into the shame and guilt that you already feel.

You should right now focus on yourself and not your ex, but the good thing is that you have informed him. Also, it sounds like you need a new doctor. Sounds like you need a second opinion. I take Valtrex once every day and I have the cream, which is effective. You also need to educate yourself more on meningitis as it is a very serious disease.

Just*in Time: May 2014

May 29, 2014

**Just*in Time**

by Justin B. Terry-Smith

**Hello Justin,**

**It has been a while. I want to say congrats on all the wonderful things happening in your life. On another note, I would love your opinion on something. When should someone like me, who is positive, disclose that information to someone you like or may be interested in? I find myself in such a hard space. Do you think guys are more open to dating men with HIV?**

**I hope to hear from you soon!**
**—Quinton**

This question is asked time and time again by all of us who are HIV-positive, unconsciously, or consciously, whether we are talking about disclosure at work or play. You might not know this, but you ask this question to yourself more often than you think.

When I was dating, I was very open about my status. It was one of the first things that I disclosed to my potential partner. If the guy that you are seeing does not want to be with you after you tell him, then he is not worth your time. Also, if he does not respect you for telling you in the first place, my opinion is to lose his number quickly. If he cannot respect you for telling him something so sacred, then he is not even worth the dirt under your fingernails….if there is any!

I have been rejected before when disclosing and luckily, I had enough self-esteem to say, "NEXT!!" For instance, I was on a date with a guy and it was going really well. At the end of the date, he and I made our way to my apartment in SW Washington, D.C. He asked if he could come up and I told him about my status. He immediately told me to get out of the car. After that moment I told myself that I would be upfront with my HIV status, even before the date started. It is better to know what you are going into instead of being blind.

One fear that a lot of us have when being HIV-positive is being rejected. Being loved, despite what the masses say, is what every human being on this earth wants. Sometimes it does not have to be love from a spouse or boyfriend—it can be friends or family that soothe or scratch that love itch we all have. The cliché that love is all we need rings true.

Your next question is a good one, "Do you think guys are more open to dating men with HIV?" Ten years ago, I might have said "no." HIV has given us time to think: If we had a partner with a terminal illness would we be okay with being or staying with them?

Also, thinking about how HIV is contracted also presses the community to question its own fear and stigma. Nowadays I think that the world, especially those within the gay community, has gotten more and more comfortable with dating people who are HIV-positive. When HIV was first discovered, it killed within years of some diagnoses. But in this day and age people who are HIV-positive are living healthy lives. If the man that you are dating is educated enough on HIV, he will know that there is a recent finding that says, in the U.S. and Canada, a twenty-year-old HIV-positive adult can expect to live into their seventies if on antiretroviral therapy. Last year, a European study found an average life expectancy for a person living with HIV was 71.5 to 75 years. Also, another recent study says that when an HIV-positive individual is considered undetectable they cannot transmit the virus. Now this is not to say go out and have sex without a condom; what I am trying to say is take care of yourself so that your virus can become undetectable. Also, still use a condom because there are other sexually transmitted infections that you have to worry about like hepatitis, syphilis, gonorrhea, chlamydia, etc. If he knows these things, then he knows that there is little risk for you to transmit anything to him.

Just remember, you have to start loving yourself before you can even think of having love in your heart for someone else. I hope this helps in your journey to find love. Also remember to take your time—good things happen to those who wait.

**Just*in Time**

by Justin B. Terry-Smith

**Hey dear**

**My name is Eric, and my family is from Jamaica. I have been positive for about eight years now. I am not proud of it, but I just wanted to tell you. Well, when I tell people they almost always compliment me on how good I look. I just tell them that I take good care of myself. I go to the gym, stay active, take my vitamins, and take my HIV medications. I used to be able to get my medications for free when I lived in Antigua but now I cannot. They are so expensive here and I am only here for a couple of years, but I am thinking about moving to Canada. I just wanted to give you a background of me and my life. But I do have a couple of questions. There are reports that say HIV is a conspiracy and that we are giving our money away to government and drug companies that just want to get rich off of us. They do not care about our wellbeing at all. Have you ever heard of David Crowe?**
**—Eric**

Well, well, well…yes, of course, I have heard of David Crowe, but many of my readers probably have not. So, let me introduce him, shall we? He is what we call in the HIV activism and advocacy world an HIV denialist. Since denialism has more of a negative spin as a label, they want to be called dissidents now. But it does not matter what they are called—they are denying that HIV causes AIDS.

David Crowe's movement has done many a disservice by spreading his movement of denialism. The denialist movement has been known to go into nations that are not well educated on HIV. By doing this they are able to influence government officials into thinking that HIV medications are only toxic to the body and do not help with managing patients' HIV. Crowe has traveled to many places, especially Africa, where he continues to spread his opinions about HIV. A lot of denialists do not believe that HIV is even a sexually transmitted disease. They believe that it can be treated by a healthy diet and exercise. Honestly, yes, it does help to manage your HIV by exercising and eating right, but it is not the only thing you have to do.

Taking your medications is very important and I know firsthand how hard it is to have to take them every day. They can be very expensive, but I would rather take my medications every day than have my body and mind wither away because I decided that I did not want to take care of myself. If you want to stop taking HIV medication, I cannot stop you; all I can do is advise you to take them and see your doctor on a regular basis.

HIV is NOT a conspiracy; the real conspiracy is someone spewing lies to other nations or groups of people to be able to take advantage of them. This is something that needs to be addressed; David Crowe and his followers have cost many people their lives, especially in countries that do not have a lot of HIV education. These people who blindly followed Crowe are not able to see that there are other options. Crowe is wrong and, in my honest opinion, he should be jailed for the thousands of lives he has affected.

Eric, I have to warn you that I have seen friends deny the fact that they have HIV and decide to stop taking medication. My friends were my age and are now dead. I have to say that, if you go down this path and stop taking your medications, there is a high probability of HIV overtaking you and turning into AIDS. Also, the chances of you being touched by more non-AIDS-defining illnesses are greater than if you were to stay on HIV medication. And I do not want that for you or anyone.

Just*in Time: July 2014
August 8, 2014

**Just*in Time**
by Justin B. Terry Smith

**Justin,**
**You know that you can reverse HIV with juicing?**
**—Fruitarian Zombie**

Ummmmm, wow, so sorry to tell you this, but that is incorrect. If this were the case do not you think that everyone would be cured of HIV by now?

I get a lot of e-mails asking or even advising me that I can cure my HIV if I just eat right and exercise; this is false information. If this were the case, I can say wholeheartedly that everyone who has HIV that wants to get rid of it would exercise and eat specific foods to get rid of it. If it were that easy everyone would do it.

I think researchers have probably already explored this cockamamie option. But there are benefits—eating right and exercising can help your body bounce back from being sick and can help make your immune system stronger; however, this does not get rid of HIV.

As of right now there is no known universal cure for HIV/AIDS. There are several things an HIV-positive person has to do to live a healthy lifestyle. Keeping your doctor's appointments: I see my doctor every three months. He requires me to take a urine test to test for miscellaneous things like my sugar levels, etc., and blood test at every visit to make sure that my viral load is undetectable, and my T cells are stable. Eating healthy is key to make sure that things like cholesterol are kept in check; some of the HIV medications may cause those levels to rise. Taking your HIV medications at around the same time every day (and not with alcohol) is also key as your body tends to adjust and gets used to you administering the medications to it.

So just juicing it up is not going to get it, honey—there is so much more than that. BUT I must say I do love my strawberry banana smoothies.

**Justin,**
**There is a specific reason why the highest risk group for contracting HIV has always been gay men. I am not making that shit up—that's fact. Look at every study. Since [HIV's] inception gay men have always been the highest contractors of HIV. HIV is a behavioral disease—it is not a sexually transmitted disease. IDIOTS!**
**—JR Munoz**

Ohh, gurl, have not we said a mouthful this morning. Well, let me give your ass a little history lesson. Gay men have been present at the beginning of the HIV epidemic, but it has nothing to do with "behavior." The death of millions has more to do with mentalities toward certain groups.

People and politicians started paying attention to the HIV epidemic only when heterosexuals started getting the disease as well [through sexual transmission]. Gay men and intravenous drug users were being infected but nobody cared because they were already looked down upon. President Reagan did not even respond to the HIV epidemic until after thousands of Americans and other people around the world had died.

Mentalities that look down upon gays is why we have had such a hard time with HIV/AIDS. HIV stigma only perpetuates fear and hate.

As you stated, "Since its inception gay men have always been the highest contractors of HIV." If a minority has constantly been looked down upon, having no rights that the majority of citizens have, made to feel like their life or lifestyle is wrong, ostracized by society, and are in some parts of the world jailed and killed for being who they are then, YES, OF COURSE THEY ARE GOING TO HAVE A HARD TIME!

Studying Public Health, I have learned that the more a target demographic feels bad about themselves the more susceptible to disease they are, and that can go for any minority that is put down by a majority.

That is also the reason why there are so many gay HIV activists who are willing to share their stories and lives with the world. Let this be a lesson to you.


Just*in Time: August 2014
August 31, 2014

Just*in Time
by Justin B. Terry-Smith

**Justin,**
**I have a question regarding PrEP as a way to prevent someone from contracting HIV. Can**

**a poz male who wants to have kids with a HIV-negative female on PrEP have children without passing HIV to her and the kid? I know of the protocol before PrEP was approved by the CDC, but what about after they approved it?**
**—Ruben Bermudez**

Thank you so much, darling, for this question. Many of my readers may not know what pre-exposure prophylaxis (PrEP) is. According to the CDC (2014) one way to possibly prevent HIV infection is for people who do not have HIV (but who are at substantial risk of contracting it) to take a pill every day. The pill, which is named Truvada, contains two HIV medicines combined, named tenofovir and emtricitabine, that have long been used in combination with other medicines to treat HIV. Now, however, Truvada is also indicated as a prevention tool. When someone is exposed to HIV through sex or injection drug use, these medicines can work to keep the virus from establishing a permanent infection. (For further information, log on to www.cdc.gov/hiv/prevention/research/prep for further information.)

Basically, PrEP is used when there is a one partner who is HIV-negative and one who is HIV-positive. This medication is used so that the HIV-negative person does not become infected when having sex without a condom (though the CDC is not advocating condom less sex). Simply put it is a new preventative measure used to decrease incidence of HIV in high-risk groups, such as sex workers, sexually active MSM, and couples, both gay and straight, where one is positive and one is negative, among others. By the way, when the news broke that Truvada would be made available, many in the gay community had already known about the medication.

If one is put on this medication, one must remember to see his or her primary care physician every three months to not only to get checked for HIV exposure but also to be checked for any damage to the liver or any organs. Remember, our bodies were not meant to be medicated for a long period of time; sometimes even medication can leave wear and tear on the body.

Now, back to your question, which can be very tricky, but I am very glad you asked it. The partner who has HIV has to have had an undetectable viral load for six months or more and is adherent to HIV treatment. There is great evidence that shows that, through adherence to HIV treatment, one can have an undetectable viral load, greatly reducing how infectious a person is. Also, some physicians suggest that, if you are thinking about doing this, you have condom less sex with the female when she is ovulating. Now some physicians might suggest that one use post-exposure prophylaxis (PEP), which is another prevention tool but a little different from PrEP. PEP is a short course of anti-HIV drugs that are meant to prevent HIV infection and administered at the earliest time possible after exposure to the presumed HIV infection.

Now back to PrEP…We must be very careful and not jump in the deep end without testing the waters first. I am a supporter of PrEP and I think it will help greatly in the decrease of HIV infections around the world. But we have to make sure that we keep in the back of our minds that PrEP does not protect against other diseases, such as chlamydia, gonorrhea, herpes, and hepatitis viruses. Condoms seem to be the other sure thing at the moment to protect humans from both HIV and other STIs. One thing is that future parents might want to be aware of that carrying other STIs leads to a greater risk for unborn children to carry them as well. Do not get me wrong—I am not saying, do not conceive if you have an incurable STI; I am just saying take the proper precautions.

Know, too, that there are other methods for mitigating the risk of HIV/STI infection during conception. My husband and I are planning on having two more kids, and if we do surrogacy, I have volunteered to be the bio-dad and my sperm would have to be sent to a facility to be cleansed then sent back down to us, where another agency would have to find a willing surrogate to carry our child, then fertilize her egg with my sperm. Simple, right? Not really, but parenting is one of the most rewarding things a person can do.

Being HIV-positive is no longer necessarily the obstacle it once was—now, you can be a bio-parent.

Just*in Time: September 2014
October 13, 2014

**Just*in Time**
by Justin B. Terry-Smith

**Hey Brother! XOXO**

**I have a couple of questions I hope you can answer about the American legal system as it relates to screening and treatment when it comes to living with HIV.**

**A friend/past dalliance of mine who is living with HIV is in Washington in jail. Word got out he is there, since April, on charges that were reportedly a set-up. However, that is not proven yet.**

**But it seems the story was released here to damage his business and reputation, by people who do not like him. It was a well-kept secret; even the government and consular officials did not know. So now the cat is out of the bag, and I can ask questions.**

**Q: I hear he is getting his meds, but what are the consequences in prison for people with HIV, in the Washington area?**

**XOXOX**
**Canadian IML Brother**

I am so glad to hear from you and I hope all is well. Let me start off by saying that it is really hard to tell someone how prisoners and/detainees are being treated because each state is very different, but I am glad you asked about just one, and I am guessing you are asking about Washington state since you are very close to it.

As far as I know there are no consequences for inmates who are living with HIV in prison, but there are challenges. The Centers for Disease Control and Prevention (CDC) (2014) states that inmates in jails and prisons across the United States are disproportionately affected by multiple health problems, including HIV as well as other sexually transmitted infections (STIs), tuberculosis (TB), and viral hepatitis.

**Treatment:**

I looked up treatment as far as the Washington State Prisons system and HIV treatment is concerned and I found some information from the U.S. Department of Health and Human

Services (HHS) (2014). According to HHS, prisons have two main methodologies for dispensing medications to those who are on ART.

The first method is called directly observed therapy, or DOT. This is where the inmate or prisoner goes to the medical unit or pharmacy for all HIV medication doses; dosing is observed by staff members.

The second method is called keep-on-person or KOP. KOP lets prisoners/inmates to keep their medications in their cells and take them independently. Monthly supplies are obtained at the medical unit or pharmacy.

Which method is better?

In 2001 Dr. Margaret Fischl et al conducted a study correlating DOT vs. KOP inmates and found out that a higher percentage of DOT patients achieved undetectable viral loads compared with the KOP patients (eighty-five vs. fifty percent) over a forty-eight-week period.

**Basics:**

According to the CDC (2011), before September 2007, the Washington State Department of Corrections (WADOC) only provided HIV testing to inmates on request. In September 2007, WADOC began routine HIV opt-in screening in which inmates were notified that HIV screening would be performed during the prison intake medical evaluation if they consented. In March 2010, WADOC switched to a routine opt-out HIV screening model in which inmates are notified that HIV screening will be performed unless they decline.

In my opinion I believe that all HIV-positive people, whether in prison or jail, deserve the respect of being able to get proper healthcare. I know a lot of people are asking, "Well, Justin, how do we pay for that?" I honestly do not know. But I know if I were falsely or legally imprisoned (and since I am a black male, I believe that has a greater chance than happening to me than my white counterparts), it would be unfair for someone to deny me my HIV medication. There is nothing more wretched than watching someone die and having the means to stop it.

Just*in Time: October 2014

October 30, 2014

Just*in Time

by Justin B. Terry-Smith

**As a father I want to have open communication with my son about HIV/AIDS and other sexually transmitted infections (STIs). A couple of nights ago while he was working on his homework, he saw me working on my column. He asked, "What are you up to Dad?" I replied, "I'm working on my HIV Advice Column." To my surprise, he quickly asked, "Is it okay if I ask you a couple questions?" So, I said, "Ask away!" So, Mr. Lundyn Terry-Smith, this column is dedicated to you, my son….**

**Dad, where did HIV come from? What was the first case of HIV?**

Well, son, that can be a little complicated. There are a lot of theories out there as to where HIV came from, but I will tell you what I know. There is a theory known as the "Hunter Theory," in which scientists have dated HIV back to the early 1900s. The Hunter Theory explains HIV via animal to man transmission. When hunters in Central Africa were hunting chimpanzees, they did not know that the chimpanzees had something called simian immunodeficiency virus (SIV). The hunters had often cut themselves, while cutting a chimpanzee's body. Since SIV is transmitted through blood, the hunter would often get SIV because chimpanzee's blood would get into the hunters' cuts. The hunter's immune system would be able to fight off the virus, but in some cases SIV would mutate into what is now called HIV in humans. This is the theory that I believe in because it has the most scientific facts to back it up.

Here is a brief rundown of some of the other more persistent theories floating around:

**Contaminated Needle Theory:** The theory is based on HIV infections from contaminated needles from human-human interaction. Basically, Lundyn, it is almost the same at the hunter theory above—just with needles. Since needles were costly there may have been an instance where a medical person would have used one needle for two or more people. Using the needle on the HIV-positive hunter first, then using it again on others would spread the virus as well….ehhhhh… it could happen.

**Conspiracy Theory:** HIV was manufactured by the U.S. government to kill off gay men and African Americans….Ummm, not the best theory, but people actually believe it….

**Colonialism Theory:** When Africa was being colonized, a lot of the colonial governments were very harsh. Often, natives became poor because they were isolated from the rest of society and were not given resources to live in the best way possible. Sanitation was often an issue and SIV-infected chimpanzees were often used as food. Also, SIV-infected needles and prostitution were rampant as well, creating a lot of chances to become HIV infected. Not my favorite theory, either.

When HIV was first discovered in the mainstream it was thought by epidemiologists that a flight attendant named Gaëtan Dugas was the first patient to have contracted and transmitted the disease in North America. That later on was found to be false. Then, through genetic testing, it was found out that the earliest case in the Western Hemisphere was a Haitian who may have worked in Africa.

In 1969 Robert Rayford, a teenager in St. Louis, Missouri, died and doctors did not know why. Eighteen years later it was discovered that he had been infected with HIV. In 1968, Rayford was admitted to a hospital with a severe infection of chlamydia, for which he was treated. But then the next year his condition got worse and he died. Since Rayford had not traveled to the major metropolitan areas, such as Los Angeles, New York and/or San Francisco or even outside the United States, scientists who studied the case in the 1980s concluded that HIV had been present in the United States before his initial infection.

Africa, particularly sub-Saharan Africa, has the highest HIV infection rate in the world. There are many countries in Africa that lack resources to be able to stop new infections. Hopefully with new medication and scientific know how HIV infections will soon decrease significantly.

Just*in Time: November 2014

November 30, 2014

**Just*in Time**

by Justin B. Terry-Smith

**Justin,**

**Let me ask you something—maybe you can put this in a blog or something…. [Here's what I want to say to someone I am seeing:] "I link you to [health] services and push you to go, so that you can know your HIV status and get screened for other STDs. We both continue to fuck around raw with other people and share our experiences openly. But when I check up on you and your health status, you continue to tell me that you have not gone, and you do not care to go. Should I continue to want to sleep with you?"**

**Is it hypocritical of me to be concerned as I also continue to fuck bareback, but I always get screened for STDs?**

**—R&B**

First, I would like to say we no longer call them sexually transmitted infections (STIs), but rather sexually transmitted diseases (STDs).

But back to your question: "Should I continue to want to sleep with you?" Honestly, wanting and needing are two different things, and wanting someone or needing someone are different, as well. If the individual you talk about is your partner or someone you aspire to be your partner, that is, someone you want in your life, I would make sure that individual cares about his or her own health. I have always said to myself: Before anyone can care for another, he or she must first care for him or herself.

When asking someone if he or she has seen a doctor sometimes you can see why the individual has refused. For example, he may not be used to seeing a doctor. But most times you cannot see why because it is psychological. He may be denying that he might have exposed himself to HIV or another STI.

As for you, all I can say is no one here is a hypocrite, but you must be careful about STIs. You are an adult, I gather, and you must take your own health into consideration. I cannot and nor do I want to tell anyone what to do with their own bodies. You need to make sure you empower yourself in protecting your own body and, in doing so, you protect others around you. If you want to continue seeing him then keep the lines of communication open. If you do not keep talking to him about being tested, he probably will not ever bring it up again, though constant communication will help, and the advice may even eventually sink in.

Helpful Hint: Sometimes I think my son never listens to me even when I tell him something until I am blue in the face. Sometimes he listens better when it comes from different people telling him the same thing.

**Justin,**

**I got tested Friday for HIV; I got my results today and they are positive. I did not know who to reach out to but you; I have followed your journey for years and now I have it, which is still shocking. I am kind of depressed. I go in tomorrow to have more labs done. I also educated myself on the laws behind it and I am determined to find out who gave it to me because I believe they knew. I have a question: Can your CD4 levels or anything show about how long you have had it?**
**—Carrie**

First thing is first: XOXOXOX. I know that feeling sweetheart.

If you want to know who infected, you that is your personal choice. There is no test that will tell you when you were infected with HIV. Also, when trying to pinpoint the person who infected you just remember he might not know that he has HIV. Do not forget—it takes two to tango. We need to remember to blame the virus, especially if neither party knew he or she had HIV in the first place. Finding out who infected you can turn into a witch hunt and become vengeful. I have seen too many times people who are put in jail even when they do not even know they have infected anyone else. I would advise that you sit down with all your past sexual partners and tell them. Just like you, they have the right to know.

Just*in Time: December 2014

December 30, 2014

**Just*in Time**

by Justin B. Terry-Smith

**Justin,**

**I do not know if this is okay to ask you, but I want to ask you anyway. We are friends on Facebook, but we have never talked. I know you add people who you do not necessarily know but at least know of your work, and that is all good with me. I am even friends with your fan page and the Justin's HIV Journal page, so I feel like I know you already.**

**Anyways, okay, have you heard of the new HIV prevention method that is a shot and shows a 100-percent efficacy rate? With all the things you have accomplished do you think you would prefer to be HIV-negative knowing that you may not have been so successful if you were negative? Also, would you take an HIV cure?**

**—Poz Swimfan**

Umm, WOW, these are all great questions, and all are very loaded. But let us take one question at a time.

If any of my readers do not know, earlier this year a new HIV vaccination method now in clinical trials with macaques has thus far proven to be 100-percent effective in preventing transmission of a hybrid of simian and human immunodeficiency viruses. This proof-of-concept study is being led by researchers at the Aaron Diamond AIDS Research Center at Rockefeller University in New York. If this prevention method is approved it would only have to be taken about three times a year vs. the currently approved pre-exposure prophylaxis (PrEP) pill, which has to be taken almost every day; is ninety-two-percent effective (in preventing the transmission of HIV), though some say ninety-nine percent; and is recommended with the use of condoms. With this new method, the shot lasted about five to ten weeks on average in the monkeys who were given the prevention candidate. My opinion: It is one step closer to a cure, at least hopefully. The more and more we come up with vaccines for disease, the more and more there is a chance for a cure. I truly believe that one day there will be a cure; and yes, sometimes preventative vaccines come before a therapeutic cure.

Now, onto your second question. A really good friend said to me that I had never looked better in my life before I was diagnosed with HIV. HIV made me change my mentality on how to live my life as it is very hard to face one's self in the mirror when one only sees pain, well I have to do that so that I can strive to live for a better life. I do have to attribute HIV with helping me refocus on what was and is important to me, which is my family, education, and health.

HIV has, I will admit, given me a degree of success, but that only came after tapping the strength I had in myself to overcome HIV and other personal demons. I used to do some things that I would normally not do to get away from the pain I would feel. I then met someone who helped me through and had me believe in myself again and what I could do to help people. My children's book helps children deal with their own disclosure, my column in a Baltimore newspaper helps the local community, and this advice column helps others around the world with questions about HIV/AIDS. If it were not for HIV, I would not be able to help others as much as I have. But who knows—if it hadn't been HIV it might have been something else?

Most of us believe in some sort of higher power, and some of us are atheist. I personally believe in a higher power and all I know is that my higher power will get me through, whether the end is near or far. I take comfort in leaving my mark here on earth, being a husband, father, and trying to be the best person I can be. So, as you can see, it is really not about my success but contributing to the success and empowerment of others that I take joy in.

Would I take the cure?

I do not know.

Just*in Time: January 2015
January 29, 2015

### Just*in Time

by Justin B. Terry-Smith

**I came across your video on the OraQuick In-Home HIV Test. I took this test three times after my possible exposure. My risk was getting a blow job from a HIV-positive woman from Africa. The whole act was about five minutes with no ejaculation. I took in-home tests on the following days after sex with these results:**

**• 84 days: Negative**

**• 102 days: Negative**

**• 126 days: Negative**

**I heard that the test has a high rate of false negatives. Is that true?**

**Do you think I can trust that I do not have HIV with these results?**

**I am asking because I have been having some weird symptoms from seven weeks after exposure non-stop up till today, about nineteen weeks later. The symptoms are tingling and pain in muscles and feet, headache, feeling like my body is overheated, fatigue, feeling ill, etc. I do not want to take a blood test here because I am in a small town in the Midwest where racists are everywhere. (I am an African American.) Sorry to trouble you, and please respond back. Thank you.**

**—Niko**

Thank you so much for e-mailing me. Let me first thank you for being proactive in your own health. I stand by and believe in the OraQuick In-Home HIV Test just as long as you know where to link to and receive resources in case the test comes up positive. Note that OraQuick provides a toll-free and confidential 24/7 support center at 1 (866) 436-6527 that will link you to services, and it also has resource finders on its Web site.

Back to your question about false negatives: Investigators found that ninety-two percent of people who are HIV-positive received a positive test result. This is called the "sensitivity" of the test. The researchers also found that 99.98 percent of the people who were HIV-negative received a negative test result; this is called the "specificity" of the test. All in all, I think that you can trust the test, but keep in mind that it takes up to a little over three weeks for HIV antibodies to show up in your system and thus for HIV to be detected by a rapid test. (An RNA test can detect HIV much earlier, but that is not a usual test unless you make a point of telling your physician that you believe that you have been exposed to HIV.) So that is why I usually advise someone who is sexually active to get tested once every three months, so therefore you have your bases covered. Also, when you do go to your primary care physician for a check-up, it is best to see if you can get tested for everything else. I know you do not want your doctor to test you for HIV, but you have to keep in mind the sexually transmitted infections (STIs) other than HIV. Your "weird" symptoms might be the result of something other than HIV, but you will not know without consulting your doctor.

Let me first start by saying that, yes, I consider oral sex a form of sex in which bodily fluids are exchanged. However, the risk of HIV transmission through oral sex is much less than that from vaginal or anal sex. In this context, the riskiest practice is performing oral sex on an HIV-infected man, with ejaculation in the mouth. According to the Centers for Disease Control and Prevention, there are also some factors that might increase the risk of HIV transmission during oral sex, such as oral ulcers, bleeding gums, genital sores, and the presence of other STIs.

Now that I have answered your basic questions, and since the New Year is coming up, I am going to ask you to make a resolution to yourself. Your New Year's resolution, should you choose to make it, is to get tested every three to six months using whatever method you would like. This means that you have to start getting tested as a part of your personal regimen.

Now I understand you are in a small town in the Midwest where mentalities can be different, not just based on race but other factors as well. But keep in mind the important thing is your health—not anyone's opinion. I would suggest finding a doctor in another town or at least stick with the OraQuick test. I know you are scared, but I would use a calendar strategy. Mark on your calendar every three to six months that you need to order the test, to make sure you do not forget.

February 13, 2015

**Just*in Time**

by Justin B. Terry-Smith

**How can one such as yourself who is HIV-positive dare to be proud of it? How do you promote unsafe sex practices being an HIV activist? Your delusions of grandeur are appalling and apparent. You tell people to be the example, but you are not setting the example yourself by being so open about your HIV status. Nobody wants to hear about HIV anymore anyways; Ebola can affect anyone, not just gays like HIV tends to do. And, yes, HIV is a homo disease.**
**—Precious Lee**

Well, hello, Precious!
What a fitting name for such a pristine young woman (I will not call you a lady). But listen up and listen well: What I do

not promote is unsafe sex. I have never said that I am proud to be HIV-positive, but I have always said I am proud to know my status. By doing this publicly I thought it might help and somewhat comfort other people and encourage them to want to know their own HIV status.

What I do promote is risk reduction when it comes to HIV. Other than trying to bash you back with unintelligent insults let us try to educate the uneducated. I am not trying to be offensive, but I am going to guess public health is not your expertise.

Since I started promoting pre-exposure prophylaxis (PrEP), which is a pill that reduces the risk of human-to-human HIV transmission, many people asked how I could not promote condoms. PrEP has been shown to reduce the risk of HIV infection in people who are at high risk by up to ninety-two percent, while latex condoms are approximately ninety-eight to ninety-nine percent effective in stopping the transmission of HIV. I PROMOTE BOTH but we HAVE to understand that we cannot tell people what to do with their bodies. All we can do is advise and tell them the facts.

Facts are sometimes scary and hard to swallow (no pun intended), but honesty hurts; sometimes the faster you swallow the easier it is to take (again no pun intended).

Any disease present anywhere on this earth is a problem whether they do a little or a lot of damage to the human body and mind. Whether it is Ebola or HIV it does not matter; they are both diseases that need to be stopped. Spending energy that is negative does not help anyone— all it does is tell everyone you have nothing better to do.

Researchers and doctors are trying very hard to keep Ebola from infecting the HIV-positive population in Africa. Even though presently there is not a HIV vaccine, numerous vaccines against Ebola are now starting human clinical trials and are being fast-tracked.

The only reason why say HIV is a "gay disease" is because in the beginning only gay men were being infected by HIV, so they named it Gay Related Immune Deficiency (GRID). When heterosexuals started getting infected by HIV, they stopped calling it GRID.

So, Precious, I hope that this intelligent response was able to answer your very upsetting questions and comments. By the way, just to let you know: How and why I can and will speak on HIV is because I have been doing it since 2003. Also, just so you know, I was recently awarded my Master's in Public Health and I landed a job (at the same time) as a Global Public Health Analyst for the Department of Health and Human Services. I am also going to attempt to earn my doctorate in Public Health. So, I tell you this, I do have the authority to speak on HIV and I will—with every fiber in my being. Nobody tells this black gay HIV positive, husband, father, author, activist, and advice columnist to sit down.

If you, yourself have not positively contributed to the world it is my personal rule and opinion that you are the one who should sit down and shut up.

**Just*in Time: March 2015**

**April 4, 2015**

**Justin—**

**Question 1: What are my chances of being resistant to anti-HIV medications? They say that it is extremely rare, but there is a chance. So, I was wondering if you would be able to answer that question for me and answer more questions. Let me know.**

**Question 2: I should be able to take a 1 a day pill. But I found out my CD4 count came back at 309. It is low. Ugh. Damn. But it should go up to at least 500 in a month if you change your diet and work out every day, right? Will that help? I will be happy if I can see it skyrocket to 900, minimum.**

**Question 3: I feel bad for the people who have to take that shot two times a day. Are the side effects of that shot really bad?**
**—The Newly Diagnosed DA**

First of all, I am going to need you to count to ten and remember to breathe! LOL.
Those are perfectly normal questions, especially for someone who is newly diagnosed.

Let us start with your first question and thank goodness it is an easy one with an easy answer. I do not know the chances of becoming resistant on those meds…but this is what I do know. There are certain things we need to investigate before we have the answer to your question. The way we find out HIV drug resistance is through testing a person's genotype and phenotype, which honestly should have been done immediately after you were diagnosed. Genotype testing looks for particular genetic mutations that cause drug resistance, while phenotype testing directly measures a patient's HIV in response to particular antiretrovirals. Until those tests come back, we will not know what your resistance is to any of the HIV medications you mentioned.

Let us tackle your second question about increasing your CD4 cell count. My CD4 count was 290 before I started HIV medication. My doctor and I decided to wait a little bit before putting me on medications. I am unsure about what my viral load was, but I believe it was 175,000. Everyone who has HIV is different; therefore, the virus acts differently in everyone. Presently my CD4 count is about 500 and my viral load is undetectable. With that being said, changing one's diet and working out every day is good for everyone. When you have HIV, it does help your body to stay fit and helps your immune system stay healthy and strong so that your body can manage your HIV and whatever other ailments that might come your way. Also, setting goals are all well and good in one's health but do not set them too high. A 900 CD4 count might be doable for some and not others.

Now, for your third question, about Fuzeon, which is injected into the body twice a day. As you may or may not know, it comes as a powder that has to be mixed with a liquid.

According to the Fuzeon website, Fuzeon can cause serious allergic reactions. Symptoms of a serious allergic reaction with Fuzeon can include troubled breathing, fever with vomiting and a skin rash, blood in your urine, swelling of your feet and/or injection site reactions (ISRs). And almost all people get injection site reactions with Fuzeon. Reactions are usually mild to moderate, but occasionally may be severe. Reactions on the skin where Fuzeon is injected include itching, swelling, redness, pain or tenderness, hardened skin and/or bumps (lasting about seven days).

Fuzeon's possible side effects include pain and numbness in feet or legs, loss of sleep, depression, decreased appetite, sinus problems, enlarged lymph nodes, weight decrease, weakness or loss of strength, muscle pain, constipation, and pancreas problems.

I hope I have been able to answer your questions. Contact me anytime. I know it is hard when you first hear the news that you have HIV, but I think that you are going to be fine. Since you are asking about HIV medication, you are curious about your health and where to go from here, instead of giving up.

Just*in Time: April 2015

**Just\*in Time**

by Justin B. Terry-Smith

**Justin—**

**So, there is a new strain of HIV from Cuba that is resistant to all known medications. Do you feel that this is a huge risk now that we have opened relations with Cuba especially for naysayers of condoms? And people who intentionally seek to become infected?**
**—Wolf Carver**

First let me inform my readers what this whole thing is all about.

It was reported in mid-February by several on-line and newspaper sources that there is a "new" HIV strain that was found in Cuba. The Miami Herald reported that the HIV strain, if left untreated, will progress to AIDS in three years. Scientists at Belgium's Catholic University of Leuven are concerned that people who are infected with the aggressive HIV strain will not at first seek treatment, and, by the time they try to seek treatment for their HIV infection, it will be too late.

First, let me say that the strain is not new (the strain has previously been found in countries in Africa), though it is rare.

...THIS STUDY WAS ONLY DONE WITH NINETY-FIVE PEOPLE, WHICH LEAVES A

LOT OF SCIENTISTS AND RESEARCHERS SKEPTICAL OF THE METHODOLOGY.

While researching just about anything in public health, we, as experts, always make sure that we have enough data from which to establish or deduce noteworthy and substantial findings for the patient populations, like the thousands of people in Cuba living with HIV, that we represent. For example, this study was only done with ninety-five people, which leaves a lot of scientists and researchers skeptical of the methodology that was used. Seventy-three patients in the study were recently infected with HIV. Twenty-one of the seventy-three patients were not classified as having AIDS, but the remaining fifty-two patients were. Those patients were then compared with twenty-two patients whose HIV had progressed after living with the virus for three years. Additionally, the study also did not consider how the subjects in the study contracted HIV.

According to the Miami Herald, Hector Bolivar, a physician, and infectious disease specialist with the University of Miami Miller School of Medicine, said, "The only thing now is that in Cuba, it is associated with rapid progression [of the disease]. It's something that hasn't been seen before that clearly."

Bolivar also noted: "It's very difficult for us in the United States or Europe or many places where there are treatments [for HIV] to replicate these findings in the long-term because it's unethical to wait until someone progresses until they can no longer benefit from treatment."

With that being said, let me first say this. Every now and then we hear of a new HIV superbug that is resistant to HIV treatment. We cannot add to public hysteria without knowing the facts through research and science. Knowing the facts is key. Then and only then will one know how to prevent infection of others and safeguard themselves from infection of not only HIV but of any illness. There will always be a risk of being infected with a sexually transmitted infection (STI) while having sex, unless we all decide to be abstinent (which we all know there is no way in hell, at least for my ass….literally).

Honestly, Wolf, whether this was happening in Cuba or Japan or any other country, there is always a risk. All in all, I really do not think it matters.

Looking at your question about the opening relations with Cuba, I cannot help but think of the HIV travel ban. Frankly, the question disturbs me not because you asked it but because other with political power might use this as an excuse to try to bring it back. If I were HIV-negative or positive I WOULD NEVER SUPPORT SUCH A BIASED LAW.

As for your second question, people who intentionally seek to become infected, which are also known as bug chasers will find a way to become infected with HIV. It honestly is not up to us to tell anyone what to do with their own bodies; all we can do is give them advice on what their options are. I personally think there are deeper issues with bug chasers than people would like to admit.

**Justin:**

**I have been diagnosed with HIV and I do not know much about what is going on, what to expect. I am not on medications yet; I am terrified of even catching just a cold and I cannot really talk to anybody because nobody knows. I mean, who is going to want to date me? —CP25**

**Philadelphia, PA**


Well, I am guessing the book, What to Expect When You are Expecting, is not the advice you were looking for, but I will do my best to help you as much as I can.

Okay, dude, first things first. You are going to be okay. I know you are horrified, but you will be fine. To tell the truth, a person with HIV can take a longer time to get over a cold, but you will probably not die because of a cold. With the ways that science and medicine are going a cold will not be the nail in your coffin. I honestly have not been sick in a long while; the only time I get "sick" is when the seasons change and that is only because I have allergies. When you get a cold, you are going to have to take care of yourself just as much as you did before you were diagnosed with HIV.

You said you have nobody to talk to about your diagnosis. I see that you live in the Philadelphia area. I must say that there are many resources that you can take advantage of. I advise that you find a support group so that you can talk about your feelings because there are a lot of emotions when one is diagnosed with HIV. Support groups are usually facilitated by volunteers and staff who are supervised by mental health professionals. Some of the groups hold weekly meetings for people affected by or infected with HIV/AIDS, their family members and loved ones. They are supposed to be confidential to keep your identity private. There are challenges that you are facing and are going to face as a person living with HIV that only others living with the virus are going to understand.

Think about this as the beginning of a new life. Even though it may not seem that way now, trust me, the more you think about it this way, the more and more positive-minded you will become about your situation. Now is the time to take better care of you. Listen to your doctor; remember, just because you are diagnosed with HIV does not mean that you have to go on medications immediately. I was diagnosed in 2006 and I did not have to go on medication until 2008.

Now here is the thing about dating while being infected with HIV: You have to keep in the back of your mind that you are bigger than HIV. There is a good chance that you might be rejected because of your HIV status. Do not worry about this; if the man rejects you because you have HIV than he is not worth it. Your main goal is hearing the "in sickness and in health" vow, right? Well, think about it this way: If that guy ever marries someone, that someone might be asking for trouble because if he cannot deal with sickness now then he might not be able to deal with it from a mate who gets sick with old age. Besides, now we have PrEP and condoms, so if they cannot deal with you being HIV-positive they are not worth your time, especially if they refuse to educate themselves about HIV and the wonderful preventative measures that we have in this day and age.

Try the organization called ActionAIDS; it is Philadelphia's largest AIDS service organization. ActionAIDS provides case management, financial services, counseling, support groups, prison services and advocacy to HIV-positive people. For more information about the organization, log on to: www.actionaids.org.

You are going to be okay—trust me. There are plenty of people around to help you through this.


Just*in Time: June 2015

June 5, 2015

**Justin—**

**Question: What would you do if you were in a situation and you needed HIV care and all the places, you are calling are telling you they are overbooked and cannot take any more people at the time. How would you address this?**

**I also have another question. Did you hear about a law that passed in South Africa that requires all people who test positive for HIV to get a tattoo that conveys this fact?**
**—Brian Edwards**

Let me address your first concern. Being in the Washington, D.C., area, it is hard for me to fathom how such a thing could happen. I would like you to think about this issue as a challenge that we should meet head-on, as some of us who have HIV-positive are in areas that are less able to care for patients living with HIV. If you are very concerned about your own health, as I am, do everything possible to sustain it. Look at which state has the best healthcare for me. See if you can afford to move to seek the care you need.

I know this may not be easy. Some people have resources to be able to get a job where they would like to live. If you do not have those resources, use your networks to look for a job so that you can move to a place that might help you better than the state you currently reside in.

I have never heard of a place that it so booked that they were never able to take me in as a patient, or a state where there are no other providers that you can turn to be able to get proper healthcare. Keep searching, baby, or find another place that will better serve your needs.

Honestly, a person's health should be paramount on the list of priorities. This is our life we are talking about here and it should be taken seriously.

Now for your second question. OMG (Oh My Goodness) I personally do not know if this is a hoax or not, but I did some research on the story. So allegedly the South African president, Jacob Zuma, has signed a provocative law that would make sure that any South African who tests HIV-positive will not only be able to access counselling and medication but will also be marked with a permanent tattoo near or around their genital parts to warn their future intimate partners. Giving people who have tested positive access to counseling and medication for HIV is a great thing but forcing them to get a permanent marking on themselves is wrong! I personally do have a tattoo on my body that does signify that I am HIV-positive, but it was because I wanted to, and it is an extremely personal choice and symbol to me.

South Africa has already had its troubles with HIV, and this would only perpetuate those same issues. Branding someone because they have an illness/disease is wrong. It will only make the general public scared to get tested for HIV because of fear of being branded permanently with an unwanted tattoo. Therefore, nobody will want to get tested and the disease will spread faster than before. It is hard to get people to do something that would benefit them if you are going to penalize them for doing the right thing. South Africa has had an issue with HIV since it was first discovered and due to political issues; past leadership has held on tight to HIV denialism and stigma to fuel their own personal agendas.

If this is a hoax, this is horrible—the most horrible hoax I have heard of in a long time. It is so personal to me and millions of others that are HIV-positive around the world.

Just*in Time: July 2015

**Justin—**

**I have to get lab work done because I am pregnant, and it is also a requirement to get an HIV test, but I am scared to find out my status. I never had any signs of symptoms of HIV, and always fight off disease pretty good. But in my past, I had unprotected sex with a couple of people.**
**—Shakira (not the singer!)**

As a parent, I have always been very straightforward with my kid, even when he does not like it. I am also straightforward with those who write in. Why? Because we as a people must live in reality to move forward in the world.

Your reality right now, Shakira, is that you are pregnant, and you need to get all the blood tests, especially HIV, to make sure that you and your baby are and stay healthy. I know you are scared about what the result is going to be, but you cannot be scared about anything until you are certain that there is anything to be scared about.

If you are HIV-positive, then the earlier you know you are the better off you will be. If not for yourself think of that beautiful life growing inside you; it lives because you live.

And do not try to self-diagnose based on symptoms; some people who have HIV might not have any symptoms whatsoever and the disease might still be progressing toward an AIDS diagnosis. It is better to get tested.

By the way, National HIV Testing Day was on June 27, but any day is testing day. Take a trusted friend with you as you get tested; you are in a delicate stage in your life and need the support. Good luck!

**Justin:**

**Ok so right now I am on no meds my T-cell count is 624 and load is 20,000. They gave me Complera, but I am scared to take it…did you experience really bad side effects? Three months ago, my T-cell count was at 908 and viral load was 10,000…the changes in numbers scares me. Sorry if I am rambling. I just wonder how long I can go without meds. Thanks for responding.**

**—Darlene**

No worries. I am on Complera right now. You have to at least try it to see if your body does well with it. If your T-cell count is dropping and you are under advisement of a doctor than you should listen to your doctor and see if it is well worth taking Complera. (I do not believe in holding anything back from my readers, so I am going to suggest you read up on it to learn about its full profile. You can start here: www.complera.com.) Complera is a great HIV medication that is fairly new. For me personally there are no side effects that I feel today. It was a lot easier with Complera because it is only one pill a day. I used to be on a three-pill regimen that included Norvir (one pill), Truvada (one pill), and Reyataz (one pill) and then I was put a four-pill daily regimen which included Norvir (one pill), Truvada (one pill), and Prezista (two pills). Now, on Complera, my T-cell count has increased while my viral load is undetectable. You have to remember to take it with food and take it at the same time every single day.

Everyone's body that is infected with HIV deals with it differently. I cannot ethically tell you it is okay to go off your HIV medication. I myself try not to miss my medication, though we all fall short sometimes. I really think you should talk to your doctor about your concerns and also going off your medication. I would not advise it, but you will do whatever you want to.

Try not to worry—the more you worry the more stressed out you will become. Living with HIV, you have to make sure you try not to stress yourself out. The stress might affect your body in combination with taking a new medication. Write back and update me about what you decide.

Just*in Time: August 2015

August 31, 2015

**Hey Justin—**

**This is the first time I have written to you so please forgive me if I ramble. I started PrEP because my boyfriend is HIV-positive, and I am HIV-negative and plan to stay that way. I am black and he is white, and our friends are a reflection on us. What I mean to say is that we have a diverse group of friends.**

**I went to my doctor right after PrEP came out and he and I talked about it. We both agreed that going on PrEP would be a good idea for me. At first, I had some stomach pain when I went on PrEP the first time, but it subsided. I think of myself as an educated man and knowledgeable about PrEP, but there is something I do not understand. Why is it that it seems Black gay men are not being educated on PrEP?**

**—Educated Black Man**

My fellow educated Black man; you pose a very interesting question. In public health we often accidentally think that one advertisement is going to work for all communities. But this is not always so.

When PrEP first came out, public health professionals made sure that it was geared toward the target population, gay men and men who have sex with men (MSM). The reason why is because these groups have higher HIV incidence rates than a lot of other populations. Public health professionals who work in the HIV field must find places where Black gay men and MSM frequent, so that they can disseminate information on public health issues, causes, information, etc.

The lack of PrEP education may be due to limited resources. In major cities information on PrEP might be more available because of the resources that that city has.

But leadership is key when it comes to spreading the word about PrEP. We have to also rely on community leaders of certain demographics to come out in support of PrEP. The reason why is because those same community leaders are exampling that people follow and some or most of them are advocates for change in their own communities. Their communities also trust those community leaders more than they trust anyone else who tells them about or how to prevent a public health issue.

Let me take this opportunity to not only suggest something not only to you, Educated Black Man, but all Black gay men and MSM that are on PrEP. Now is the time for you to become community leaders. The more and more that you speak to the Black gay and MSM community the more information they are going to be able to get the information that they need on PrEP, thereby protecting themselves from HIV. A lot of people will not do this because they are scared of the stigma that is associated with taking PrEP.

Fuck that and fuck PrEP stigma. But, honestly, you have noticed a hole—now fill it (no pun intended). By hole I mean the one in the public health arena. I have always had a high respect for anyone who sees an issue and does not merely talk about it but puts a plan of action in place. I do not know you at all, but I think that you might want to seriously take some time and think of what it would mean to your community if you came out as an Advocate/Activist for PrEP. I am not sure what state you are in, but if this is the path that you want to go down, then I suggest contacting a local and more powerful non-profit that is advocating for PrEP. Get information from that organization on PrEP and begin to ask places if you can disseminate information. This is your community, and it needs you. We must all band together to stop the stigma that stifles our community to create a healthier tomorrow.

We need to be able to step up and stand out. Finally, I will leave you with these very wise words from the civil rights activist and another Educated Black Man, Bayard Rustin: "We need, in every community, a group of angelic troublemakers."

September 24, 2015

**Hey Justin—**

**I am Samuel, but you can call me Sam. Okay I know you probably get a lot of questions e-mailed to you but thank you for reading. I first heard of you when I read your column for Baltimore Gay Life newspaper and now, I am loving the advice column "Just*in Time"; it is such a great resource for people living with HIV.**

**I have been living with HIV since I was eighteen and now, I am twenty-five living strong. I made my first speech as a person living with HIV a couple years ago and it felt really good. Speaking of years back I remember you were on Norvir, Truvada and Reyataz at one point in time. How did you like that medication? Did you have the gel caps for Norvir? When traveling how did that go with the gel caps?**
**—Sam**

Well, let me say thank you first and foremost for following my work. It is really important that activists and advocates in the public health field are able to reach the population, thus influencing policy and people's mindsets about certain populations and illnesses. Speaking out as a HIV-positive person can be therapeutic and empowering for the one speaking and at the same time educational for those that are listening to you.

Since 2010 the Food and Drug Administration (FDA) approved the tablet form of Norvir to be prescribed to those who need it. Since then, I honestly do not know anyone who is on Norvir that still takes the soft gel tablets, unless they have not told me yet. Now I am on Complera, which is a one-pill-a-day regimen. I like it a lot.

Sam, keep on speaking to the people; they need to be educated on HIV and as long as there is no cure then we need to keep trying to prevent HIV incidences, especially in countries that are not as developed as others.

**Justin—**

**Hey, sexy Justin, I am a future adult entertainer, and I am a little scared. I am seeing more and more adult movies coming out that are geared toward bareback sex. Do you think this is true? I was always taught that bareback sex was bad. What is your opinion on barebacking?**

**—Future Adult Entertainer**

First, thank you for the sexy compliment. To bareback or not to bareback is a decision we all have to make on our own. As a public health professional all I can do is tell you to weigh your options. If you decide to have bareback sex and you have tested negative, I suggest you talk to your doctor about pre-exposure prophylaxis (PrEP). As you might know the CDC has stated it is about ninety-percent effective in preventing HIV infection between one person and another.

In the past the community and myself were anti-barebacking. People who barebacked were often looked down upon and were basically slut-shamed, which is detrimental to any population. If that is not what you are into, who are you to tell others what to do with other consenting adults? It is really nobody's business. My opinion on barebacking is that as long as you and your sexual partner(s) know the risk and are okay with them, who am I to try and stop you?

The adult industry has seen its multiple scares of sexually transmitted infections (STIs), even though they do try to safeguard their workers from HIV and other STIs. But sometimes YOU must take the initiative and safeguard yourself, especially if you are going into the bareback adult industry. I myself admit that I watch bareback porn and I do not look at any of my friends that do bareback porn any different than my friends who are adult entertainers that do not. We should not judge the men and women who are in the adult entertainment industry; in fact, I was once a stripper and an escort, and I do not mind telling my story. Just remember to take responsibility for your own health on either path you take.

Just*in Time: October 2015

by Justin B. Terry-Smith

October 22, 2015

**Hey Justin—**

**Can I ask you something about STDs? I am from Turkey, so my English is not so good.**

**That can lead to death, right? Sorry 4 asking. I am just so scared about that thing. Please message me back as soon as u read my message. Thanks.**
**—Noel**

Thank you for your question. Well, I would need to know what STD you are talking about. (Also, we are trying to not say STD anymore we try to use STI or sexually transmitted infection, as this helps decrease stigma for people who live with STIs every day.)

Now, let us start with early detection; early detection is paramount when dealing with any STI. The earlier that you find out that you have an STI the more options you will have to deal with the STI itself. Any STI that you let linger inside your body will only get worse. Most STIs have cures but some only have options to suppress the STI.

Here is a list of curable STIs: chancroid, chlamydia, crabs, gonorrhea, scabies, syphilis, trichomoniasis, yeast infection, vaginosis, and yeast in men.

Here is a list of incurable STIs, but I will go into more detail about them.

Hepatitis can be very tricky, because there are five types, and they are hepatitis A, B, C, D, and E; some are curable, and some are not. Presently, there is no cure for hepatitis A, B, or D, though there is a vaccine for hepatitis A and B. There are new drugs that cure hepatitis C that been shown to cure hepatitis C at an effective rate of ninety-five percent. Hepatitis directly affects and damages the liver. There is no cure for HIV/AIDS. HIV is the virus that causes AIDS, but with medication can be suppressed to the point where someone can live just as long as someone without HIV. HPV/Warts, which is an infection on the genitalia and a women's cervix, are also cureless. Herpes is a common disease that can present itself in the mouth (cold sore), anus, vagina, and/or penis. Herpes presents itself as a blister on the regions of the body listed above.

Whether or not a STI is curable or incurable, the important thing to remember that it is you who has control over what you do next. I have friends who are co-infected with hepatitis and HIV, and who continue to live long healthy lives. But to live a long healthy life one must make certain provisions to one's own lifestyle. I have been living with HIV for ten years and I have made provisions, but I also fall short in some of them. When I was diagnosed with HIV nine years ago, I was a wreck, I did drugs and drank entirely too much. I decided to make a change. I started running three miles regularly and working out when I could find the time. I also changed my eating habits. Since the medication I was on made my cholesterol increase I needed to change my diet. So, I do not eat pork as much and I decrease my egg intake. I started eating more and more fruit and started shopping for more low fat and low sodium foods. I may not be the epitome of good health, but I push onwards and upwards.

Having an incurable STI is hard, but it does not mean you should give up. Once you are defeated in the mind, your body will follow and falter. It is not the end of the world, but it is another reason why you should live your life healthier than before. There are incurable diseases in the world and some we may not even know about yet; and on that note, I will leave you with these famous words by Nobel Prize-winning biologist Joshua Lederberg: "The single biggest threat to man's continued dominance on this planet is the virus."

Just*in Time: November 2015

by Justin B. Terry-Smith

November 25, 2015

**Hey Justin—**

**Does PrEP give you a false sense of security that you can engage in more risky behavior, such as bare sex for instance?**

**It has to a certain degree, but I would say no more or less concern than before I started taking PrEP. Before PrEP, I had very few sex partners and I knew my HIV status and my partners knew their HIV status. We were all negative. We would not use condoms because we were in our minds safe and being responsible by getting tested regularly and limiting**

the number of guys, we had sex with regularly. My doctor asked why I was getting tested every three months (the window of infection) for HIV. I explained that I had a couple of sex partners that I was having bare sex with and wanted to be sure I knew my status at all times.

I personally feel nothing with a condom on and cannot maintain erection to completion. It is very frustrating and that is the real reason I chose bare sex with limited partners. After talking to one of my sex partners who just went on PrEP and explained it to me, I went back to my doctor and brought PrEP up in conversation. He immediately thought I was a good candidate for it and should go on it considering my confessed sexual activity.

My doctor surprised me by saying that undetectable HIV-positive men were likely a better sex partner because they were on meds to block it and I was on PrEP to block HIV, too, so the likelihood of contracting it was very low, versus having sex with a guy who thinks he is HIV-negative but is in fact positive and highly infectious. Since that talk, I am less apprehensive about engaging in sex with poz undetectable men, so I guess the answer would be yes. I do feel more at ease and probably have a false sense of security, but at least I am proactive and taking PrEP to provide a barrier against HIV. I no longer am afraid to love someone who is HIV undetectable and no longer afraid to have sex with them.
—The Chad

Thank you for writing me. I do not believe that it does give you a false sense of security; whether or not you engage in risky behavior is based on whether you make that decision, PrEP or not. One of the concerns for researchers and activists is that PrEP will give people an excuse to engage in riskier sexual behaviors. According to Guest et al (2008), the overall sexual risk behavior did not increase during a PrEP trial. The number of sexual partners and rate of unprotected sex acts decreased across the twelve-month period of study enrollment. The data also indicates that the HIV prevention counseling associated with the trial was effective.

Good for you for being tested and having open communication with your sexual partner and your doctor. This is a prime example how many of us should be talking to our sexual partner(s) and physicians. I agree with your doctor on how it might be easier to have a partner who is HIV-positive, but love is love and attraction is attraction—you cannot control that. But if you do get involved with someone who is HIV-positive and on medication it might help with adherence to PrEP as well. According to Ware et al (2012), if one partner is on PrEP and the other was also taking medication (ART or cotrimoxazole as prophylaxis against opportunistic infections), they might match their own dosing schedules to their spouse's, as a way of promoting adherence (for both).

---

**References:**

Guest, G., Shattuck, D., Johnson, L., Akumatey, B., Clarke, E. E. K., Chen, P. L., & MacQueen, K. M. (2008). Changes in sexual risk behavior among participants in a PrEP HIV prevention trial. Sexually transmitted diseases 35(12), 1002-1008.

Ware, N. C., Wyatt, M. A., Haberer, J. E., Baeten, et al. (2012). What's love got to do with it? Explaining adherence to oral antiretroviral pre-exposure prophylaxis (PrEP) for HIV serodiscordant couples. Journal of acquired immune deficiency syndromes (1999), 59(5).

Just*in Time: December 2015

by Justin B. Terry Smith

December 21, 2015

**Hello Justin—**

**My name is Alex, and I am a twenty-six-year-old gay, HIV-positive man. I live in Oklahoma and I have always known I was gay since I was a boy. Well, growing up in Oklahoma was hard so I moved to the big city this summer. I was like a kid in a candy store dating and having sex with men.**

**Then I found out I was HIV-positive a month ago and my world came crumbling down on me.**

**Then I met a beautiful man who became the light in my life. He swept me off my feet, we took things very slow at first and I loved every moment of it. When I say I loved every moment of it, I mean that getting to know him before sex was great.**

**When I felt comfortable, I told him I was HIV-positive and he did not seem to mind, except for when we tried to be intimate. He says it is not me, but I think he is not telling me the whole truth. He is not able to get hard when I want him to perform anal sex on me; we have done everything and anything to try to get him ready to have sex with me anally, but it still does not work. The only thing that seems to work is giving him a blow job and he usually "finishes" that way, too. Please help me; I think that I might have found the one, but I want to be able to satisfy him and vice versa. Please tell me what to do.**
**—Alex**

Hey, Alex the Great. Thank you so much for writing in. This is something that I have heard before from others who have e-mailed me. I say, do not worry or panic. First, let me just say trust is a big issue for a lot of couples. Sometimes men get scared and do not want to admit it to their partners. I would ask him, "Have you ever been intimate with anyone before me that was HIV-positive?" His response might give you more insight about whether or not it might be because you are HIV-positive or because he might need a little assistance getting hard.

Oral and anal sex have very different sensations and feels, and the tip of the penis is very sensitive and much more sensitive with lubrication. But all in all, you see where I am going with this…at least I hope you do. It could be that he enjoys oral sex more than anal sex because of the way it makes him feel physically.

I would suggest that you both might want to sit down and talk about how it makes him feel physically and find out why he might like it better than anal sex. I am not a sex therapist but would love to be. If you cannot talk about it alone with each other I suggest seeking the help of a sex therapist.

My next suggestion would be to go to a doctor and find out if he or she would recommend or prescribe some "assistance" for your partner. In my opinion this situation is reversible in a good way. I had an ex who needed the little blue pills for ED, but after we were together, he did not need them. It turns out that being HIV-positive had nothing to do with it.

Even though being HIV-positive can affect not only us, but our loved ones, as well, to better fight stigma we need to have an open dialogue. We need to be able to open up about our fears and concerns. You need to stay strong because either way there is going to be work that needs to be done on both of your ends. Hmmmmm I think I did mean to say that…lol…hopefully you are both versatile. Signing off, with love and lube.


Just*in Time: January 2016

by Justin B. Terry-Smith

January 21, 2016

**Hey Justin—**

**I saw a post you did in Facebook about apps and dating sites and it caught my eye because I was on Adam4Adam.com. I was on the lookout for a hook-up and I am HIV-negative. I kept seeing these profiles that said, "On PrEP." I did not understand, and I was wondering if you could help me.**

**I do not understand why people would want to use a pill rather than use a condom. Can you help me understand that? I want to know what your thoughts about going on PrEP are, because, Justin, I am really scared. I have been used to using condoms for years and I am a single father, and I do not want to put myself in jeopardy, possibly losing my life, because I want to be there for my son.**

**—B Right**

First of all, I want to say thank you for having the courage to write to me; I really appreciate that you are confiding in me with your information and concerns. Let's be PrEPared for 2016!

Being a father is really hard and being a single father is very hard, but I am going to try to prepare you for 2016 the right way. I am a father of two gay boys who are seventeen and nineteen years old. I have assisted my nineteen-year-old in obtaining PrEP, or pre-exposure prophylaxis, a relatively new prevention tool based on taking the

anti-HIV medication Truvada, because my husband and I have decided to make him responsible for his own health. He had a boyfriend at the time, and he wanted to go on PrEP because he had heard about the benefits of it. I love my son to death, and I want him to be able to protect himself as much as possible. I did feel a little indifferent when putting him on PrEP but, as his feelings are the ones that count most, I was glad because he was being proactive about his health. Each one of us has to learn what preventative measure is the best for ourselves. I was worried, of course, because being on PrEP is a very hard thing to do because it is outside of the norm that we are used to, but ultimately, I was glad that he was aware of his options and in control of his choices.

You, too, have this choice to make. Many people go on PrEP because the feeling of having sex without a condom is better because of the feeling, which is okay. But we have to be aware that PrEP does not protect against other sexually transmitted infections (STIs), such as hepatitis and syphilis. And, according to the Centers for Disease Control and Prevention (CDC) (2015), PrEP is up to ninety-two-percent effective in preventing HIV transmission among those who are considered to be at high risk (sexually active MSM, for example). These are issues that we need to understand and to be aware of, but I will say here and now that I am an advocate of PrEP.

Though PrEP is relatively new, we need not to be scared of new preventative measures. Many people of an older mindset are asking people to be wary of PrEP, which they should be. PrEP, like I said before, is not a preventative measure against other STIs. The only reason why people are so scared of PrEP is because people do not understand things that are new and innovative.

So, let us get down to the nitty gritty. You know PrEP is taken once a day, every day. You need to be adherent to PrEP for it to remain optimally effective. PrEP does not fight against any other infection except HIV. There is very little evidence that PrEP has the same serious side effects as seen in positive individuals on Truvada, though long-term studies on PrEP use by negative individuals have yet to be conducted. Remember, if you go on PrEP take the pill early in the morning or afternoon so you do not forget to do so. Talk to you doctor and listen to him/her.

---

To read the Centers for Disease Control and Prevention information, log on
to: www.cdc.gov/hiv/prevention/research/prep.


Just*in Time: February 2016

February 26, 2016

**Justin—**


**We have been friends (on Facebook) for a while and we met [as fellow members of] the leather community when you were Mr. Maryland Leather 2010. However, I would appreciate it if you keep my identity secret, seeing as how we are both well known in the leather community as well.**


**Well, I noticed that there is a spike in syphilis cases among gay men, especially in the leather community. Do you think that has anything to do with pre-exposure prophylaxis (PrEP)? My next question is about post-exposure prophylaxis (PEP). In your opinion do you think that PEP gives people permission to have sex with others and then go get the pill the next morning?**

**—Old Guard Leather DADDY**


Thank you for writing me and forgive me for responding a little late. Since Mid-Atlantic Leather Weekend just happened, I have decided to use your e-mail as the one that I want to showcase for this column.


Recently, there have been surges of not only syphilis but other sexually transmitted infections (STIs) in the United States. According to the CDC (2015), in 2014 there was about 20,000 cases of syphilis that were reported. That was the highest rate since 1994 and a fifteen-percent increase over 2013. The CDC stated that 458 cases of syphilis in newborn babies; this has been about a 27.5 percent increase since 2013. There were also a reported 350,000 cases of gonorrhea, which is a five-percent increase since 2013. The CDC is also saying that researchers have found that those individuals who are taking PrEP for HIV prevention did not contract HIV; however, some did contract gonorrhea and syphilis. I should also note that some researchers are saying that syphilis is being better reported and that is why the number of infections is so high.

I do not think we should stigmatize people because they choose to use PrEP or PEP. Let me first describe to my readers what PEP is and then what PrEP is.

PEP is an anti-HIV drug that should be taken as soon as someone thinks they have been exposed to HIV. PEP is only effective if taken within seventy-two hours of exposure to HIV and it must be taken for twenty-eight days. It consists of two to three antiretroviral medications. It is not a simple regimen as you make it seem—it is not one pill the next morning.

PrEP is a once-a-day medication taken specifically to prevent HIV, which is ninety-two-percent effective. Neither PrEP nor PEP are 100-percent effective in preventing HIV infection between humans. PrEP and PEP are both preventative measures that we need to make sure that the general population know about, including when and how to use them.

Also let me say this that there is no study that says that there is an increase of syphilis in the leather community. But let me say this: The early AIDS epidemic started right at the beginning of the sexual revolution for the gay community. People do not understand that that is one of the reasons why our community has such a big problem with HIV/AIDS. We were asked to suddenly adapt our freedom to a new situation, and we were also increasingly stigmatized. We had to fight for our lives. Former President Ronald Reagan did not even say the word "AIDS" in a public speech until thousands of people had already died. Also being gay in the eighties was not easy because we were so looked down upon; nobody gave a flying fuck about our community, except us and our allies. We went through years and years of burying friends every week. I was born in 1979 so I never did see the tragedy of the early AIDS epidemic, but my friends, especially my friends who are gay and men who have sex with men of color, are still dying.

I would like to pose a question to my readers if they would not mind sharing their opinion. With the rise of PrEP and PEP do you think that the gay community has the ability to relive their sexual revolution or has the gay community already been there done that?

March 24, 2016

**Justin—**

**Quick question. Since you can still get the other STDs, can HIV hitch a ride on those when they are transmitted?**
**—Vernon**

Hey, thank you for replying to January's installment of Just*in Time. This is a very good question, and it is a question I have never gotten before. But let me analyze the question before I answer it. I am guessing what sparked your question was that I spoke of in the last column, which was about PrEP and how someone who is taking PrEP is still susceptible to other sexually transmitted infections (STIs).

PrEP is highly effective in preventing HIV, period. As far as what the research says, STIs cannot act like a Trojan horse and smuggle in HIV in the presence of PrEP.

But to answer your question about the relationship of HIV and STIs in a general sense: YES, it can go either way. If you have the human immunodeficiency virus (HIV), you can leave yourself open to other STIs; and if you have an STI, you can leave yourself open to HIV.

Let me explain further so everyone understands what I am talking about. The transmission of HIV and STIs are highly similar. If a person becomes infected with HIV, they may have put themselves at risk for other STIs such as chlamydia, hepatitis, gonorrhea, herpes, syphilis, etc.

With some STIs you are at greater risk of being infected with HIV. STIs, such as herpes and syphilis can cause open sores on the body. These sores allow HIV an easier pathway to introduce itself into the body through the bloodstream. Even though STIs such as chlamydia and gonorrhea primarily do not show themselves with symptoms of open sores, they still leave the body to be more susceptible to being infected with HIV. When the body becomes infected it sends CD4 (cluster of differentiation 4) or helper cells to the infected area to help stop the infection from spreading. But that makes it easier for HIV to introduce itself into the body by attaching itself onto the CD4 cells. Once HIV has attached itself to these cells it will have the ability to infect them and travel throughout the body. So, when a person is showing symptoms it is best that a physician check for HIV and vice versa.

Also, there is an interesting fact that I found in my research, which I already knew but did not think of. If someone is HIV-positive and they are infected with another STI, such as herpes, his or her symptoms can be more severe. Herpes is an STI that will on occasion show itself through sores on the infected part of the body, such as the anus, penis, vagina, mouth, or even face. Seeing as how HIV directly affects the immune system, being co-infected with herpes leaves the body open for more outbreaks of herpes than there would be if there was no HIV infection in the body.

If you are already HIV-positive you can also be more infectious to others if you are co-infected with other STIs, such as chlamydia and gonorrhea. Seeing as how the body sends more CD4 cells to deal with the STI co-infection it gives HIV more of a chance to infect more CD4 cells, thereby giving HIV the ability to spread more easily throughout the body. Therefore, when an HIV-positive male is co-infected with another STI, such as gonorrhea and chlamydia, the HIV viral load in the semen increases. BUT when the STI is treated the HIV viral load tends to decrease.

In conclusion we have to all remain vigilant about taking care of ourselves and understanding the signs that something might be wrong. Do not ignore signs of infection because you could not only be protecting yourself but protecting loved ones as well. One of the things that I wish to see in my lifetime is one pill that protects against all STIs, something like PrEP but on a universal level. Science and medicine are amazing when they have the ability to work together and work together well. Hopefully, the future will see more collaboration and more strides in fighting against HIV and STIs.

Just*in Time: April 2016

by Justin B. Terry-Smith

April 27, 2016

**Justin—**

**This is in response to the expected HIV infections in the Black Gay population that I saw in one of your posts. It cited stats from the CDC that fifty percent of Black Men will [likely] test positive as will thirty percent of Hispanics. My question is: Are we doing the right outreach in light of this prediction and, if not, what should we be doing?**
**—Bob Doyle**

I hope all is well. I will address your question but let me further clarify to the readers just what it is you are talking about. In late February, the Centers for Disease Control and Prevention sent out a report on HIV infections among gay males and men who have sex with men (MSM) population.

Utilizing diagnoses and death rates from 2009–2013, CDC researchers projected lifetime risk of HIV diagnosis by sex, race and ethnicity, state and more. The CDC stated that if the present HIV infection rates continue on the trail that they are going, then 1 out of 2 Black/African American gay and bisexual men and 1 out of 4 Hispanic gay and bisexual men will be diagnosed with HIV in their lifetime; gay and bisexual Caucasians still have a 1 out of 11 risk of being diagnosed with HIV in their lifetime.

The release went on to say that regardless of sexual orientation 1 out of 20 Black/African American men and 1 out of 48 Black/African American women will be diagnosed with HIV in their lifetime. 1 out of 48 Hispanic men and 1 out of 227 Hispanic women will be diagnosed with HIV in their lifetime. Caucasian men and women have less than one percent chance of being diagnosed with HIV. Certain areas, such as the Metropolitan Washington, D.C. area, are and parts of Florida remain high.

Now, Bob, for the first part of your question: Are we doing the right outreach in light of this prediction? There seems to be a major disconnect between outreach on so many different levels. One of the important things to learn in public health is not to engage one community the same way you would another. The reason why is because needs across communities are different and how one population engages a public health issue may be entirely different than another. Also, for example, if there is a target population that speaks mainly Spanish, you would probably not advertise a public health program in English, with no translation whatsoever. The message has also changed from what it was to what it is now. The HIV that most remember is from the early AIDS epidemic of the early 1980s and 1990s, where many gay men and MSM, among others, were dying left and right, where AZT was the only known HIV treatment, where HIV was also known in the Black/African American community as a white man's disease, etc. The generation of Millennials and some Generation Xers (through no fault of their own) do not and cannot recall those things or images, unless they Google them, but they are not necessarily any wiser than earlier generations. The face has changed (and realize that that first face was not entirely accurate) and there needs to be a new messaging in HIV prevention, especially that which is marketed to minorities.

PrEP is now available and there has been marketing towards gay men and MSM of color, but it is not enough. There needs to be more and in a more innovative way, instead of going to night clubs that gay men and MSM of color frequent and handing out a flyer about PrEP. Messaging on PrEP also needs to be targeted to gay men and MSM of color in their own communities. There also needs to be more and more examples of public health leaders that are gay men and MSM of color on PrEP so that their communities see someone that is familiar to them and looks like them utilizing PrEP. When a community sees, hears, and feels something they are familiar with, they are usually more comfortable with it.

Just*in Time: May 2016
May 23, 2016

**Hi Justin—**

**I really like your column and I read it when you post it on your Facebook fan page. But there is something that you've yet to talk about and I want to bring attention to it, only because I may have questions about it that some others have as well. I do not live near a big city or have really great Internet connection where I live, but the subject that I was looking into is the Zika virus. It seems that it is getting more and more of a problem and it scares me. I am HIV-positive and have been for twenty-eight years. I am doing well and am thriving. But being alive during the early stages of the AIDS crisis, it scares me that the Zika virus will be the second coming of a virus that will affect the gay community. What do**

**you think? Also has anyone who is HIV been infected with the Zika virus yet? Are we as HIV-positive people more susceptible to catching the Zika virus? Please help me.**

**—Country Boy**

THANK YOU! FINALLY! I have been waiting on a question about the Zika virus for a while. Let us start by giving my readers some brief information about the Zika virus. The Zika virus is primarily spread through the bite of the infected Aedes species mosquito, which also spread the dengue and chikungunya viruses. A pregnant woman can also pass the Zika virus to her unborn child, which can cause microcephaly (a condition in which a baby's head is significantly smaller than expected, often due to abnormal brain development). At the time of delivery, the Zika virus can also be spread from mother to child.

The Zika virus can be spread by a man to his sexual partners. There are cases known today where the Zika virus has been sexually transmitted by men who have developed symptoms of the Zika virus. Researchers have found out that the Zika virus can be spread before and after the men showed any symptoms. Scientist have found that there is a case in which the Zika virus was spread a few days before symptoms developed. The Zika virus is present much longer in semen than in blood and if you have been infected by the Zika virus, you are likely to be protected from future Zika infections. The Zika virus currently has no vaccine.

In May of 2015, the first case was recorded of autochthonous Zika virus transmission in a thirty-eight-year-old HIV-infected patient who was born and is living in Rio de Janeiro, Brazil. The Brazilian researchers also have found the Zika virus in urine and saliva but are now unsure if it can be transmitted in that way.

I do think that gay men might be more susceptible to being infected with the Zika virus because one of the ways it is carried is through semen. In the case of the Brazilian patient who is infected with both HIV and the Zika virus, the CD4 count (619) and viral levels (undetectable) of HIV remained the same for four weeks after the patient was infected by the Zika virus. Presently, researchers are engaging in more scientific studies to increase knowledge of the Zika virus and whether or not there is potential of another viral epidemic. Symptoms of the Zika virus can last up to a week, and they can include fever, rash, joint pain, and conjunctivitis (pink eye).

We need to be proactive about finding more about the Zika virus and to not take it lightly. We need to protect ourselves as efficiently and effectively as possible. That protection should be based on education and awareness. In the gay community we have seen such strife and loss and do not need to have another epidemic. We need to make sure that persons in power take us seriously as not only citizens of this country but as human beings.

Just*in Time: June 2016

June 20, 2016

**Dear Justin—**

**I am in the medical field and I just wanted to say thank you for all the work you do. Even though I work in healthcare I do not have much knowledge about HIV. I have a friend that is a special friend. I met her at my office; we will call her Angela. Angela is eight years-old and her adopted mother admitted to me that she had [been diagnosed with] AIDS. I could not believe it when I heard, but the thing I also could not believe is her strength. Angela looked at her mom and said, "Oh Mom do you got to tell everyone," before letting out a long sigh. It seemed Angela was not afraid of answering question about herself either. Angela blurted out, "Yes I was born with it." I was so amazed by her but there was a sadness about it all. I wondered and asked myself if she was ever going to have a life? What kind of life would she have? But I could not figure out the answer myself, so I am asking you. Thank you for any help you can give.**
**—Sal Tofer**

Good day to you and thank you for writing in. I understand what might be going through your head. There are a lot of questions that many people would have to know to see if the child's body is handling the infection.

I am not sure if you know the difference between HIV and AIDS, but there is a difference, at least in science and medicine's eyes. T cells are helper cells that help the body fight off illness and infection. When you are infected with HIV and your T-cell count goes below 200, the doctor might give you an AIDS diagnosis. The one thing that I like to mention to people is positivity goes a long way. Angela obviously may understand her diagnosis and is comfortable with it. She might be more susceptible to infection because of her AIDS diagnosis, but she has her adopted mother who is giving her access to proper care. Also, another factor that must be considered is if her viral load is detectable. The viral load is how much HIV is in the blood. If she has an undetectable viral load, it means that there are so few copies of HIV in the blood that monitoring tests are not able to detect the HIV.

From the information you gave me in my opinion she will be okay. Even though she is very young and has an AIDS diagnosis it does not mean she is not having any kind of life. From what you have told me it seems like she is the typical eight-year-old girl. Seeing as how science and medicine and making advances in the HIV sector I am very optimistic that there will be a cure, maybe not today or tomorrow but someday, and I want to be here to see it. They are also coming out with better medications that do not have so many side effects and negative long-term effects on the body. I personally know of a man who is ninety years of age who just died from being on dialysis but did not die from HIV. He is considered a long-term survivor considering he was diagnosed over thirty years ago. I read a study that explained that a person who is twenty-five and diagnosed with HIV can live a long healthy life if they are taking care of themselves, as in a good diet, exercise, on medication, etc. When I say a long healthy life, I mean a life with a life expectancy that someone without HIV can have. I would not worry about Angela; it seems that she is being taken care of and before you know it you might be getting an invite or notification to her high school graduation.

Thank you.


Just*in Time: July 2016

by Justin B. Terry-Smith

July 20, 2016

**Dear Justin—**


**I hope you get to read this because I am in desperate need of an answer about HIV prevention.**

**I actually met you years ago when you were the speaker at Howard University for Black AIDS Awareness. I was a freshman then and I did not know a lot about HIV. I think the reason why is because I did not know how to accept the fact that I was gay. When I finally acknowledged it, I thought about your presentation at Howard University. It scared me because I did not want to be HIV-positive. I had a boyfriend and we had sex only about twenty-five times. He was very abusive verbally at first and that really took a toll on my self-esteem; then he became physically abusive and would throw things at me in the house, punching me, smacking me, etc. I left him and now I have a new boyfriend.**

**My new boyfriend is amazing, but he is also HIV-positive. He does not want to use condoms, but he wants me to go on PrEP; I kind of already know what I want to do but I really wanted to know what you would do in this situation. Do not worry—I am not basing my decision on what you say, but I am going to take it into consideration.**
**—A**

I hope all is well. I, too, have been in an abusive relationship before and I am glad that you made it out of it. As you stated, domestic violence can decrease self-esteem, thus leaving those victims more susceptible to becoming infected with HIV. That is, an individual experiencing violence may not take precautions to protect himself or herself. Sexual health may seem like the least of their worries.

You mentioned precautions in your letter, so it sounds like you are taking more ownership of your sexual health. In that context, let us talk about PrEP. PrEP is ninety-two to ninety-six-percent effective in preventing HIV transmission. If I were HIV-negative and I had my choice again, at first the decision would be hard for me. I would have to think about the benefits and the limitations. I would probably choose to use PrEP over condoms, and I would not look back. If I were in a relationship at the time, I would probably want to have a talk with my boyfriend and our doctor(s) to see what HIV preventative prophylaxis would be beneficial to the both of us.

You have to understand that I am from Generation X. We were the generation that grew up with condoms as the primary way to prevent HIV transmission. It was the preferred way, at least for me. The other way was abstinence and there was no way in hell I was going to do that. No matter what, however, taking control of your sexual health sometimes comes with struggles.

I lost my virginity to a female at thirteen and used a condom; I lost my virginity to a male at seventeen and used a condom as well. I used a condom until the age of nineteen, when I had sex with a guy that excited me enough to stop the precautions.

Then two so-called "friends" informed me that he was HIV-positive. I cried my eyes out for hours; I agonized about going back to base (I was in the United States Air Force) and taking an HIV test. I took one test when I got to base and then one test three months later and I was HIV-negative. Then days later after the three-month test, I found out it was a cruel joke, and he was not HIV-positive, and my so-called "friends" were just jealous. In a way, they were controlling my sexual health—not me.

The point of my telling you this story is to take control of your own sexual health. Whatever you choose whether it be condoms or PrEP (or condoms and PrEP), the point is that you are the one taking control. You make the choice of how you want to protect yourself and others around you. Granted, the general message is to use both condoms and PrEP at the same time, but we do not live in a reality where we can be assured that that practice will catch on. People are going to make their own choices about their own sexual health, as you have here, and as everyone else should feel they have a right to do so.

Just*in Time: August 2016
August 9, 2016

**Got a question you might know the answer to....So I am negative and on Truvada as PrEP, but my boyfriend finally got on what I thought his doctor prescribed him, Truvada, but instead was Emtriva. Now I have done my homework and before I get out of sorts: Is Emtriva equal or effectively the same as Truvada? Just thought you might know more than me, who specializes in sales and not health. Any help would be appreciated.**
**—JCrew**

First, let me commend you on taking control of your own health. By being on Truvada you are protecting yourself, as you know. Many people do not want to go on pre-exposure prophylaxis

(PrEP) because they prefer condoms only. This certainly has been a subject of contention in the HIV activist community.

Okay, let us address the issue. First, let me explain that Emtriva is utilized with other HIV medications to help suppress HIV infection in the body. It allows your immune system to work better while being infected with HIV. Emtriva also lowers the chances of an individual who is infected with HIV of getting opportunistic infections, such as a cancer-causing infection. It also reduces the risk of HIV transmission. Truvada is made up of two medications, tenofovir (Viread) and emtricitabine (Emtriva).

Honestly, I think you really need to talk to your boyfriend. Open communication is where you are going to find your answer. If you are not sure about why he is taking the medication you need to ask him. I am not a doctor, but maybe you should consult one so that you know the facts. I do know that being honest allows for couples to be able to share information that they may have been apprehensive to share if there is no open communication. I would suggest sitting down with him and making sure that you do not sound judgmental when asking about the medication. I always ask when the last time is a person has had their last HIV test because I personally do not want to run the risk of transmitting the virus to them.

The second issue would be to question why the doctor did not prescribe him Truvada. There could be a very good reason why his doctor paired Emtriva with something other than Viread. But I raise this issue because a lot of doctors will prescribe the same preventative or HIV medications to the couple in a relationship. Sometimes being on the same meds can also be a lot easier for the couple. Partner A and Partner B are in a relationship with each other; Partner A and B are both on Truvada. If Partner A runs out of Truvada, he can always ask Partner B if he can use his medication until his prescription of Truvada comes in. I am not saying this is the right way to do things, but I know it does happen in real life. One would have to be very cautious to make using another person's prescription a standard practice. Importantly, one should never just prescribe oneself Truvada as PrEP. Consult a doctor before just taking PrEP out of the blue. The same goes for HIV medications. If Partner A is taking Complera and Partner B is taking Triumeq they should not mix up their drugs because Complera and Triumeq have their differences, even though both of the medications are dosed at one-pill-a-day to suppress HIV. Consult your doctor before switching medication with your partner. The reason why I advise not to do this is because everyone's body handles different HIV medications differently. Meaning, I am on Complera because I consulted my doctor, and my body has been doing well with it from the very beginning. If I lost my pills or ran out of Complera I would not want to try to take another HIV medication to compensate. The reason why is because I do not know how my body will react to that certain medication.

My advice is not to tell you what to do, but to give you options on what to do or tell you what I would do. I leave it in your hands to make the right decision for yourself. Do a little bit more research.

Just*in Time: September 2016
September 21, 2016

**I need your help. I am writing from Ghana, where every gay person is living in the closet. I am married with kids. I recently had sex (I was top) with a guy without a condom (that was very foolish of me) who was about nineteen years-old and who I met on Facebook. A day after the regrettable act I noticed a spot of discharge in my pants; I did not take it seriously because I foolishly thought a pubic hair might have pricked the urethra and that it would stop on its own. I waited about eighteen days until I saw a doctor. My urine test showed presence of bacteria and a urethra swab showed presence of staph bureaus. I took a number of antibiotics. The discharge stopped after a day of taking antibiotics. My wife got infected in the process and was given antibiotics after a urine test and then a uterus swab and blood tests when she complained of lower abdominal pains.**

**Both of us had some headaches and fever, which were treated. I am still nursing a mild headache. I am so scared that I might have contracted HIV during this single gay sex encounter. I know I have to go for a test, but I am scared. If it is positive how do I tell my wife and ask her to go for a test too? Not a day passes without me weeping and praying that my wife should not be positive even if I am. She is a good woman and indeed the backbone of the family and the pillar against which the children lean. Please help. Do I have HIV? I have never been able to have more than a two-hour sleep in the night for about two months since this happened.**

**—Ivory**

Let me say that it is really heartbreaking that there are people in the closet because of the fear that is related to being open about who you love. Some of my readers do not know that in some countries one can be jailed or even killed simply because of stigma and fear of what people do not understand. This fear of not being able to be who you are directly contributes to increased HIV infection rates. One cannot protect oneself if one is not proud of who they are. Now let us address your problem, Ivory.

When there is a possible infection of a sexually transmitted infection (STI), I believe that one will benefit to get tested for all of them. Frequently STIs come in clusters, and, also, people do not realize they have an STI because they are not showing any symptoms. I have never heard of a headache being a symptom of HIV but that does not mean that you and your wife should not be tested for HIV. I know you are scared but it is better to get tested early. If one gets tested for HIV early there is more of a chance of survival and less chance of opportunistic infections to develop.

I cannot tell you whether you have HIV or not—the only way that you will know is if you get tested. You need to be tested as soon as possible. You say your wife is the pillar of your family; the only way a pillar stays strong is to take care of it. Also, you might want to invest in HIV preventative measures. The more traditional preventative measure is a condom. But if one is not available you might want to try pre-exposure prophylaxis (PrEP), which is a pill taken once a day that significantly decreases the risk of HIV transmission. Keep in mind that PrEP only decreases your chance of being infected with HIV; PrEP does not protect you from other STIs, such as chlamydia or gonorrhea. In Ghana researchers conducted a study on PrEP and sexual behavior. The study found that people who went on PrEP did not have an increase in their sexual activity. Bottom line—get tested!!

Just*in Time: October 2016
October 18, 2016

**Hi Justin—**
**Greetings from Accra. I cannot stop admiring your online posts and pictures and your positive attitude toward life. This makes me wonder if you are really HIV-positive because you do not fit the popular image of a person living with HIV as melancholy and lonely.**

**Most people here do not disclose and are living in silence because of stigma. This brings me to the question: How did you find out you are positive—of course it was by testing but what led you to go and test for HIV? Did you have symptoms? What were they? How long after your exposure to the virus did you get tested?**

**These appear to be personal questions. It is okay if you do not wish to answer any of them. Thanks, and regards. Good health and blessings to you.**

**—Kaya**

I hope all is well and thank you for writing in. I also want to thank you for reading my articles and posts; it really helps me to know that people out there are really reading and listening to what I have to say. Let us talk about the image of a person living with HIV. In the 1980s and '90s living with HIV was very hard. On top of having a life expectancy of five years, give or take, one's view on life could sometimes become altered. Knowing that you are HIV-positive can lead someone to depression, to become isolated and can lead others to discriminate against them, etc. These negative factors can become overwhelming and can affect how a person treats themselves as far as living healthfully—physically, mentally, spiritually, and emotionally. When there was no medication that could effectively help someone with HIV, the complications of HIV were a lot worse. But today, because of medications called antiretroviral treatments, people with HIV are able to live healthier lives, to the point where someone with HIV can live nearly as long as someone who does not have HIV. The images of HIV in the 1980s and '90s are very different than they are today, at least in the U.S.

To address your other questions about my symptoms and testing: One day I woke up and my satin sheets were soaking wet. I then began to throw up five times in my bed and realized that something was wrong. I had never felt so sick before, except for when I had the flu. I found out that I was HIV-positive because of an HIV test that I took at a local nonprofit in Washington, D.C. I was tested in 2006, but I believe I was infected in 2005. I have been living with HIV for eleven years but diagnosed ten years ago, in other words. I know there are people out there that would say HIV does not exist. Those people are called HIV Denialists or Dissidents. Do not believe them because HIV does exist; it is a scientific fact, and no legitimate/ethical doctor will tell you that there is a cure. Many doctors that say they have the cure for HIV are fraudulent and, in my opinion, they have the blood of people who believed them on their hands.

Many cultures still have HIV stigma and, today, because of stigma, people do not disclose their HIV status and are living in silence. The image of people living with HIV in some cultures is that they deserved getting HIV. They blame the victim of the infection and not the infection itself. This directly affects an HIV-positive person living in that same culture. They do not want to be associated with HIV for fear of what family or friends might think of them. Sometimes this can lead to them not seeking treatment and not disclosing to their sexual partners, thus leading to more infections and more deaths. From my experience with friends who have died in the past, there is still stigma. I went to a funeral of a friend and nobody wanted to say what he died of, even years later. That is what stigma does. Speaking out helps others accept what HIV is and helps them to combat it.

Just*in Time: November 2016

November 27, 2016

**Hi Justin—**

**I heard your dissertation is on pre-exposure prophylaxis (PrEP). Can you tell me what the side effects of PrEP are?**

**—Robert**

Thank you for e-mailing me. Currently, the antiretroviral therapy drug called Truvada is the only drug combination indicated as PrEP. Even as PrEP is becoming a driving force for HIV prevention, there are side effects to PrEP.

Public health professionals would like to make sure that we know the positives (prevention of HIV transmission) and negatives (i.e., side effects). When it comes to long-term treatment as prevention, there are long-term and short-term side effects.

While taking PrEP some of the short-term side affects you might encounter are nausea, abdominal cramping, vomiting, dizziness, headache, and fatigue. Since PrEP is a new entity to the body, it will take time to get used to it. The first-time side effects may arise is within one to two weeks of starting PrEP; the side effects also take one to two weeks to subside. Whenever you start a new medication there is a risk of short-term side effects but at least with PrEP we know that they will eventually go away.

When looking at long-term side effects we have to look at a person's behavioral factors. For example, if a person smokes, drinks, or takes recreational drugs he or she is more likely to develop illnesses and that may lead to more susceptibility to the PrEP side effects. But the basic side effects of PrEP are bone density loss and chronic kidney disease. We also have to look at behaviors that might combat the long-term side effects, such as engaging in physical activity and increase in vitamin D intake.

**Justin,**
**What did it feel like when you got HIV? Did you notice your body change? And, if so, did you think it was nothing? Or can you just not tell at all if you are positive?**
**—Aaron**

I've had a little time to think about your question. Please keep in mind I had to think back to 2006 and that was ten years ago. So, by your first question, "What did it feel like when you got HIV?" I am going to guess that you mean when I started showing symptoms. In my opinion I believe I was infected in 2005 but I did not start showing symptoms until 2006. I can remember one night I was at a night club with four of my very good friends. I started feeling warm as if I were getting a fever. I went outside to get some fresh air. When I went outside, I felt the urge to throw up and so I did but felt much better after that. I merely thought I had a stomach bug. Then a couple months later I was in my bed and woke up sick. I threw up five times and noticed that all my bedsheets were wet because I had sweated on them when I was sleeping the night prior to being sick. I went to the clinic with my best friend and that is when I found out that I was HIV-positive. My body did not change except for throwing up. The only way you can determine if you are HIV-positive or not is if you get tested for HIV. You can go to your doctor, a clinic, or buy an over-the-counter home HIV test. But I will inform you that going into a clinic you will have access to more resources if you find out that you are HIV-positive. The over-the-counter HIV test allows you to have privacy while you find out the results of the test, but the downside is that you will not have any resources at the tips of your fingers if you find out your test is HIV-positive (or HIV-negative). When I found out that I was HIV-positive I cried while at the clinic, but I had a grief counselor and my best friend for support. All in all, get tested to know your status.

Just*in Time: December 2016

December 27, 2016

**Dear Brother Justin—**

**Greetings of peace and may this letter find you well and richly spiritually blessed. My name is Asar and I am presently locked down inside of this slave ship on dry land for making an unwise choice in my life. However, since I have been here (six years) I have taken positive advantage of the many self-help programs. My biggest gain has been my earning a doctorate degree in comparative religious studies.**

**I am writing because I came across an old issue of A&U Magazine (February 2016) and I read that you are studying for your doctorate in public health. By the way, I am an HIV/AIDS peer counselor here at the prison and I am in dire need of some African-centered intervention materials. In addition, why are our people in such denial about HIV/AIDS? How do we get Black folks to deal with reality? Do our people suffer from some psychological block of some kind? Are we suffering from some kind of psychosis?**

**Maybe these questions might be the basis for your dissertation? But in all seriousness, do you have some papers that have been written by Afrocentric psychologists that deal with these issues and possible solutions to this crisis? Perhaps you know of an African-centered HIV/AIDS organization or Black psychologist that is or has done research in this area? —In Solidarity,**

**Brother Asar**

Brother Asar,

Thank you so much for writing in. Let me first start out by saying thank you for having the courage of being an HIV Counselor, which I am sure it is harder being institutionalized while trying to give hope and resources to HIV-positive clients, and I am glad you are taking advantage of the many self-help programs. Congratulations on earning your doctorate degree in comparative religious studies.

There are many reasons why African Americans could be in such denial about HIV. There is still a mistrust of the government, dating back to the Tuskegee Syphilis Experiment. The U.S. Public Health Service partnered with the Tuskegee Institute in a clinical study which enrolled 600 black men from 1932 to 1972 and violated medical and scientific ethics; 399 were infected with syphilis and 201 were not infected with syphilis ("Tuskegee Study of Untreated Syphilis in the Negro Male"). The researchers told the participants that they were being treated for "bad blood." None of the participants were properly treated for syphilis, even though penicillin had been known to treat syphilis since 1947, less than halfway through the study.

Alongside mistrust, there is also a lack of education and shaming when it comes to a person becoming HIV, as if they had done something wrong to become infected. Homosexuality continues to be condemned by the Black church; this is very detrimental since the church has long since been a steeple in the black community since slavery. The issue that might need to be addressed is acceptance and education. Once people of the black community start accepting the people who are HIV-positive or those who are more at risk of becoming HIV, then they can become educated on prevention and the detriment of shame and stigma.

We must understand that African American ancestors were once slaves and were assimilated into thinking, from a Christian confine, that anything that is different from the Bible is wrong. That kind of mentality has given our community a block to not accept or educate itself as to why we have such an issue on HIV.

Some of the helpful resources that instantly come to mind are materials prepared by the Black AIDS Institute (BAI), which is located in Los Angeles; Us Helping Us People Into Living Inc. (UHU) in Washington, D.C., and Gay Men of African Descent (GMAD) in Brooklyn, New York. I am praying that this helps you in your search for answers.

By the way, my dissertation focuses on the extent to which factors of socioeconomic, education, and numbers of sexual partners relate to the utilization of PrEP.

Shalom,

Your Black Jewish Brother

Justin B. Terry-Smith aka Yadin

Just*in Time: January 2017

January 20, 2017

**Justin—**

**Been a while since we last chatted. I am really interested in surrogacy, as I want a child of my own. As I explained before I am positive, undetectable for many years. Can you advise me where I can go to get this done at an economical cost? Based on my research there are a few organizations that do it, but I would rather get a referral than take what I hear online. Any advice?**

**—Ebenezer**

I hope all is well. I really want to give you advice, but first I would like to start out with my own story on fatherhood. Before my husband and I got married we had a talk about children. He really was not thinking about it, but I felt I had a need to procreate. So, after our talk, we decided that we would explore all options. At first, we looked at surrogacy by researching different clinics in our area. When we found one that we were comfortable with we made an appointment. We saw a doctor and mentioned that there might be an issue since I was HIV-positive. The doctor gave us options and mostly we did not like them. For instance, there is a hefty bill that comes along with trying surrogacy and being HIV-positive. So, the procedure of sperm cleansing will be very costly. Insemination of the surrogate costs about $10,000. Then you will need to make sure that the sperm has inseminated the woman; sometimes it does not work the first time, which will cost more money. At the start of the process, you must find a woman who is willing to be inseminated by your sperm. You will then have to pay for her medical expenses for the entire pregnancy. Then you have the hospital expenses, as well. All in all, there is a pretty penny to pay when it comes to surrogacy. When we were looking for a company to go to that specialized in sperm cleansing for HIV-positive men it was suggested that "some people mortgage their house to help pay the expenses." This totally turned me off to the idea. But I think you need to go through your own journey with surrogacy. Everyone has to have their own journey when it comes to parenthood.

The one solution that my husband and I came upon was going through our state's Department of Social Services (DSS). We took a training called PRIDE training, which was great and almost weeklong. It was all about the rules and regulations of adopting or fostering a child. Our house then needed to get inspected by the Fire Marshal/Fire Commissioner to make sure it was safe to have children and the DSS had to come out to the house to tell us how many children we could have in our house (depends on the size). After this was complete, we immediately got a call from DSS about a fourteen-year-old boy who identified as gay within hours of being approved because we did stipulate that we would take a LGBT youth that needed a home. Then our second son came to us because he knew of our first in high school. This is how we became parents.

Many people do not think that people who are HIV-positive can become parents. At one meeting a person asked, "How do we keep the child away from the parent if the parent is HIV-positive?" When I heard a guy ask that question, my husband had to stop me from saying something—not to mention his wife was so embarrassed. But we had to educate him on his ignorance, and so we did. Just because you have HIV does not mean you cannot use surrogacy to have a child but know that there are plenty of children out there that need a loving home. Merry Christmas, Happy Hanukkah, Happy Kwanza ,and a Happy New Year.

Just*in Time: February 2017

February 22, 2017

In this column, I have decided to address slut-shaming—trying to make someone feel bad for what is perceived as having "too much" sex or the "wrong" kind of sex. Individuals living with HIV have often been slut-shamed—according to some, we are not even supposed to have any kind of sex!

Slut-shaming is wrong in any context, but it becomes nonsensical in an era of Treatment as Prevention. I have HIV and am, thanks to anti-HIV meds, undetectable, and, if you do not live under a rock, you might have heard of pre-exposure prophylaxis (PrEP), a prevention tool for negative individuals—both fall under Treatment as Prevention, using medications to stop the transmission of HIV. If you are undetectable you have suppressed your viral load on antiretroviral medication and have long (or at least for six months) been undetectable, meaning there is a negligible, and some say nonexistent, risk of transmitting HIV, you and your partners may decide to not use condoms. If you are negative, you may decide to use PrEP as a form of HIV prevention, with or without a condom.

I was on a social media application (no, I am not telling which one) where one of the statuses you could chose to support was "Treatment as Prevention" and I did. Sometime later, I was approached by someone that had not-so-nice things to say to me because of my support of PrEP. I heard things like "You're a slut; only a whore would condone raw sex; have fun at the clinic."

After all of this negative, slut-shaming energy, I had to take a couple of deep breaths and turn it into something positive. So, I have decided that I would come up with a list for Treatment and Prevention supporters who often encounter slut-shaming in 2017. Why? Because slut shaming directly contributes to stigma. Being stigmatized can contribute to the lowering of self-esteem, which can also make people fearful to go on preventative treatment and to go on HIV medications if they have been infected with HIV. People need to have supportive networks, not stigmatizing ones, especially within their own demographic. The LGBT people and HIV community should be uplifting one another because we have enough people misunderstanding and hating us.

So, what can we do?

**There is a block button.** No matter what social media you are on, it does not give anyone the right to be an asshole. Just block them. There will always be someone who is going to find you attractive—why are you wasting time with someone that is not going to give you the love you want?

**Unfriending is not unlawful.** Look, millions of people are on Facebook and you do not necessarily have to talk to them. There are PrEP discussion groups that you can be a part for support and, trust me, they are in your corner.

**Educate them:** Yes, we must make sure that we leave space to educate those of us who judge everyone else's sexual lives. Which gives room for a lot of assholes to teach. But, with that being said, I sometimes leave a link to a website to educate on PrEP and new, innovative prevention measures.

**Slut-shame them right back:** One of the biggest controversies for people wanting PrEP was being called sluts and whores because they were being open about looking for the love that they wanted. Usually, people who have huge opinions on the sexual lives of others, have their own sexual proclivities that they do not want to share with others. (No mentioning certain politicians here.)

**Oh, I am a whore—why do you give a fuck?** I always ask people who judge my sexual appetites: "Do you want me sexually? If no, then fuck off….Next…." The real question is, why do they care?

**So, I am a Truvada Whore?!** No, seriously, I am a Truvada Whore and I own it: There are people that own it, and that is okay. The term "Truvada Whore," once meant to stigmatize, was reclaimed; it comes from a movement of empowerment. It may mean that "I'm HIV-negative but for my HIV prophylaxis I'm going on PrEP"; or "I'm HIV-positive and I would like my sexual partners to be open to or only use PrEP as a HIV prophylaxis." Some people have a problem with being called a whore and that is fine, too. We all own parts of our sexual proclivities, but the important thing is we do not judge others for their own or by a standard we have no business putting on others.

**Walk the fuck away.** No, seriously, there is more than one out there. What I mean is that you have to have the empowerment in yourself to just walk away. Sometimes when approached by someone who only uses condoms, I give a compliment and say, "I never did mind about the little things." Then look down in between their legs and walk away.

All you have to know is that it is their choice. Never mind about the insulting comment I just made in last tip; just say, "Okay thanks, but I'm looking for something different." They do not have to accept your stance, but they do have to respect it. PrEP is an acceptable form of HIV prophylaxis, but so is a condom. Your sex life is your own and so is theirs, so fuck 'em…or not.

March 31, 2017

When being first diagnosed with HIV I personally handled it as best as I could. We all handle our diagnosis in different ways. Some people become severely depressed, some look at it as a chance to live their lives in a healthier way, and some, believe it or not, are happy because they do not have to fear HIV transmission any longer. With mixed emotions flying high, we must remember some important things about not getting depressed about having HIV.
I came up with seven ways to fight HIV depression.

**Find a Network:** Networking with people of like interest is important personally and professionally. There are plenty of HIV communities either online or in person that you can join. These groups, whether you find them on online social media or face to face, are meant to help you through this process. There are people you will find that have and are going through the same thing as you are. It is important that you know you are not alone.

**Go to Events:** The community can always use help. My suggestion is first start off small. The first event I think I ever went to or got involved with was a White Attire Affair whose proceeds had benefitted an HIV/AIDS organization. Next, I decided to do the Washington, D.C., AIDS Walk/5K Run, until my knee started having issues. There are small and large events you can attend, whether you are in a small or large community.

**Join the Fight:** Become an activist and start organizing fundraisers, join HIV campaigns for prevention, or go to different organizations and ask them, "How can I help?" Volunteer for an HIV organization that has ideals that align with your own. This can help you further your own education in HIV.

**Get Political:** There are going to be several obstacles that you are going to face being HIV-positive and politics will be one of them. Some politicians are continuing to take away monies that directly affect programs that reduce the cost of HIV medications for underinsured and uninsured persons with HIV. The Ryan White CARE Act, which was first enacted on August 18, 1990, is the largest federally funded program for people living with HIV/AIDS. Congress has to reauthorize the act so that it can be extended for another period of time. Ryan White gives a huge chunk of its monies to the AIDS Drug Assistance Programs, which gives HIV medication to HIV patients across the United States. So yeah, it is kind of important that we fight for it.

**Seek Counseling:** Sometimes you just need to vent to someone about what you are going through. But I suggest trying to find an HIV counselor or ask your local HIV organization if they have counseling services. If not, ask if they can refer you to a therapist who has a specialty in HIV or infectious disease. There are also numbers that you can call to be able to talk to someone who understands.

**Find Solace in Friends:** If you choose not to disclose your status and feel that you are going to bust keeping this in, chances are it is not helping your mental, physical, spiritual, or emotional state. Try to find a friend who might understand what you are going through and who is not going to judge you based on your HIV status.

**Get Spiritual:** I know that I am really not one to do this myself, but I see that some of my really good friends that were recently diagnosed with HIV turn to their higher power or spiritual leader. A lot of them tend to feel better when turning to their own spirituality and drawing strength from it. Now whether you are a Jew, Muslim, Christian, Buddhist, etc., it does not matter—if you find strength to get through tough times by praying or getting involved spiritually, do it. It cannot hurt, try it.

Just*in Time: April 2017
April 27, 2017

Whenever we divulge our HIV status, we never can predict what reaction we get. But we all know that there are common questions that people ask. Sometimes, those questions can be personal, uncouth, and/or downright rude. I have several friends that I have known for years that do not even recognize their own ignorance and assumptions when posing their questions to me about HIV. But this is not about what is "right." This is about educating people on HIV (and maybe throwing a little bit of "shade" in there, too!).

So, this month we are going to delve into the top seven questions people have asked when revealing your HIV status and the answers that an HIV-positive individual could use as a retort.

**Question: How long do you have to live?**

**Answer:** I do not know; how long do you have to live?

Now, this question was asked by a relative and I thought it was revealing how uneducated he was. Please keep in mind that nobody knows when they are going to die. When my relative asked me this question I was about twenty-six and this was the best way I knew how to answer this question at the time.

**Question: Is the reason why you are skinny because of HIV?**

**Answer:** No, my parents just have the body of gods—what is your excuse?

Society has made it socially acceptable to be slender but that, by no means, should justify someone using the word "skinny" to describe another person. The word "fat" is used to describe someone that is outside of society's norm of what a body should look like—well, so is skinny. The word "fat" is usually used in a derogatory manner to describe someone's body, and, well, so is skinny. I do not know how many times I have heard someone describe another as "that skinny bitch" or "that fat bitch." All in all, it is wrong.

**Question: Do you tell everyone you have sex with that you have HIV?**

**Answer:** Do you tell everyone you have sex with that you do not have HIV?

I find it interesting that people are more concerned with your sex life when you are HIV-positive. But, honestly, if we want a world to have full disclosure with our sexual activities, proclivities, and natures then it must be all the way around. What is good for the goose is good for the gander.

**Question: Do you still have sex?**

**Answer:** I do not know—am I still alive? (You should answer this question while giving a side eye for effect.)

HIV-positive persons have the same sexual desires as everyone else. When I see a hot guy/lady, yes, I might get wet on both ends and my mouth might start to water, as well. Of course, sex is and will always be thought of when I see a hot person walk by. We are still alive, and we still have sexual needs.

**Question: Is you partner HIV-positive, too?**
**Answer:** That is a question you should be asking them.

I have encountered this question more often than not. But, luckily, you can throw the ball in someone else's court and keep it moving.

**Question: You are going to tell the new person you are dating that you are HIV-positive, right?**
**Answer:** When I am ready and when the moment is appropriate to discuss with them, which this is not.
Though I concur that honesty is the best policy, everyone who is HIV-positive has their own time in which they would like to divulge their HIV status to a potential sexual partner. It is nobody's business when you plan on revealing your HIV status to anyone.

**Question: There is a cure for HIV—did you hear about it?**
**Answer:** Obviously not, because I would not be HIV-positive right now.

You may get people telling you that there is a currently affordable cure that is accessible to the general population. I have gotten many e-mails stating that there is a witch doctor in Africa claiming they have a cure. I suggest deleting that conversation as fast as I delete those emails.

Just*in Time: May 2017: So, You Want to Be an HIV Activist

by Justin B. Terry-Smith

May 23, 2017

So, you want to be an HIV Activist…

There are several things that you should be aware of or put in place so that you can become a HIV activist. When I became an HIV activist, I had to keep in mind that there are different ways for one to become an HIV activist. There is a virtual activist, who is more of a present-day phenomenon; this kind of activist uses social media such as YouTube, Facebook, Twitter, etc., to spread their message. There is the more traditional activist, who will organize a protest in numbers and bodies to put up picket signs and yell slogans. In this country and world, we need both and more allies to join causes even if it does not affect them directly.

## 1. Think of the question "why?"

Why do you want to be an activist? There is a thing call passion, and most of us have it. What are you passionate about? There are many aspects of HIV that one might feel passionate about. Whether it is HIV policy change, HIV funding, prevention, awareness, or education—all are needed in this fight.

## 2. Research.

Once you figure out what part of HIV activism appeals to you, do your research on it. You have all the resources at your fingertips. Anyone can use Google to research subject matter on HIV, but there are better ways to get the latest news on HIV. Go to an HIV organization or health agency and sign up for their newsletter. Make sure that the agency does its fact-checking and that their news is accurate.

## 3. Talk to people.

Hey, I have a good question if you are not positive yourself: Do you know anyone who has HIV? If you do not now is the time to meet someone living with the virus. Talk to a person who has HIV and find out the challenges on what it means to be HIV-positive: how much their medications cost them with or without medical insurance; the big issues that are paramount to them.

## 4. PrEP or Condoms?

One of the biggest issues that HIV activism has recently faced is whether to advocate for PrEP or still stick with condoms. I, for one, advocate for both. I prefer PrEP but I also understand that condoms are acceptable as well. Condoms prevent other sexually transmitted infections (STIs), while PrEP only prevents HIV. PrEP can be used by anyone who is negative, but it has given men who have sex with men (MSM) a new and revived sexual revolution, a reboot of the one that had been stilted by AIDS. There are pros and cons to both; it is up to you to figure where you stand.

## 5. Street smart or book smart?

One of the biggest issues in activism is being well educated on the aspects of HIV. There are activists who have never gone to school to receive a higher education degree and they do not have to. Being educated on recent issues is very important, but one does not need a degree to understand what is paramount to the HIV community. But I will say that having a higher education degree can give a person more power to have the ability to travel into the different areas of HIV activism.

Remember, these are just five things you need to think about before becoming an HIV activist. There are many more things that come along with being an HIV activist. Please remember that being an activist is important to any cause. Representing an underserved community is often hard, especially when you, yourself, are a part of that community. Think about the people who you are going to help in the future because of what you are doing. Many individuals say to me, "Nothings ever going to change." I say, "Nothing ever changes for people who don't bury their head in the sand to what goes on around them." Since you are not doing anything to make a change, stop complaining about how nothing changes.

Good luck and see you online or in the streets!

Just*in Time: June 2017
June 21, 2017

**Hey Justin,**

**I know you talk about HIV most of the time and sometimes I really wish you would talk about something else. So, I figured that I would write to you so you can help me with another issue I am having. On top of having HIV, I learned that I have herpes. When I**

**went to the doctor I was not informed whatsoever. It turns out that in the doctor's office there was a magazine (A&U Magazine) with your column in it. That is how I discovered you, so can you shed some light on herpes for people that may be like me, diagnosed and not informed.**

**—Martin Hivpes**

Okay, now there are many sexually transmitted infections (STIs) that we have to be conscious of and herpes is no exception to that rule. As most of you know I tend to put a little humor in my columns so bear with me…or not; it is going to happen anyway. So, I am just going to go right into to it. Here are my top 7 things about the gift that keeps on giving that you need to understand:

## 1. Common herpes

Herpes is a very common STI and most people that have the herpes virus do not know it because they do not show any symptoms. Even though someone does not show any clear signs of having the herpes virus it can still be spread from human to human.

## 2. Types of herpes

There are two types of herpes virus, herpes simplex type 1 (oral) and herpes simplex type 2 (genital). Herpes simplex type 1 is transmitted through the mouth; this can happen through sharing toothbrushes, eating utensils, and kissing. Herpes simplex type 2 can be spread through sexual contact with another person.

## 3. Now you see me, now you do not

Herpes outbreaks can come in the form of blisters and be brought on by fatigue, stress, menstruation, suppressed immune systems, and trauma to the area of infection. To be blunt, use lots of lube and make sure you are taking your time when engaging in intercourse. Of course, we all know sex can get rough and hard; just make sure your using proper lube so trauma can be reduced at the area of penetration. When having an outbreak, do not engage in sexual intercourse. You may cause one of the blisters to rupture and that will increase the chance of herpes spreading to other places.

## 4. Cure and treatment

Presently, there is no known cure for herpes, but there is treatment. There is prescribed oral medication that comes in a pill form that has to be taken daily (Zovirax, Valtrex, and Famvir). Also, there is a cream-based prescribed medication (Acyclovir) that is to be applied to the genitals and on the anus. For oral blisters, there are several topical medications that you can get over the counter, such as Abreva. Also, women who are pregnant should regularly consult a doctor because herpes can infect their unborn child.

### 5. Avoidance issues

So, you ask how can I avoid herpes? Live in a human condom—no just kidding. Seriously, you can reduce the number of sexual partners that you have, practice monogamy, exercise abstinence, or wear a condom or another form of latex barrier while engaging in oral, anal, and vaginal sex.

### 6. If left untreated…

If left untreated in adults, herpes can leave a person more susceptible to other STI infections, such as HIV. There is also a greater chance to develop encephalitis or meningitis, bladder infections, swelling of the urethra, and rectal inflammation. If left untreated during a pregnancy then the baby can be born blind, brain damaged, or even death can occur. There have also been recent studies that show that untreated herpes might be the cause of Alzheimer's disease.

### 7. Diagnosing herpes

Consult your doctor because you can still lead a normal life with herpes. If you feel the need, ask your doctor to administer a blood test to find out if you have herpes.

Just*in Time: July 2017: Reflections on Pride
July 13, 2017

It was a typical day at Washington D.C.'s Pride parade, the sun was out, people were smiling, cheering and….protesting? When I am in the parade you can usually catch a glimpse of me in the leather contingent on my motorcycle. I live about forty minutes outside of the D.C. area, a little bit of a schlep for some. If you are in the Pride parade, in any Pride parade, you can expect some delays, but during this year's Capital Pride, there were several.

A major delay was caused by #NoJusticeNoPride, which, according to its Facebook event page, is "a collective of organizers and activists from across the District of Columbia. We exist to end the LGBT movement's collusion with systems of oppression that further marginalize queer and trans individuals." They were protesting Capital Pride for several reasons. Their demands were to honor the legacy that trans women of color played in the history of Pride by adding more transgender women of color in leadership positions; more stringently vet which corporations serve as sponsors of Capital Pride; and prevent uniformed police officers, including the LGBT Liaison Unit of D.C. Metropolitan Police Department, and military personnel from participating in the parade. They were chanting "We shut shit down" and "We're here, we're queer, get used to it."

At first, I was a little puzzled by it all, maybe because I do not necessarily identify as trans or queer, maybe because I, myself, even though gay and black, understand that how I was raised makes me privileged I am not sure. The parade was delayed for about ninety more minutes than expected, which cost the city of Washington, D.C., a pretty penny. Also, the parade was rerouted three times in order to bypass protestors who had chained themselves together in order to interrupt the flow of the parade.

I understand their demands listed above. Having representation of all of the LGBTQ community is very important in the parade. I also think that the leadership that represents us should be strong, competent, knowledgeable, intelligent, and articulate, to name a few requirements. But I do have some questions. Have they themselves come up with a better vetting system than the vetting system that Capital Pride already has in place for its sponsors? Isn't the last demand, of preventing uniformed police officers, including the LGBT Liaison Unit of D.C. Metropolitan Police Department from participating in the parade, a little farfetched, considering they are for our protection? There have been incidents when police have protected the LGBTQ community from harm during pride parades and festivals. As far as military, talk about exclusionary—I myself have marched proudly as a member of the military member, a 9/11 disabled veteran, in uniform.

I am all for raising one's voice when there are injustices, and everyone should have the right to protest. Pride itself once was a protest. The first gay marches took place in New York, Los Angeles, San Francisco, and Chicago on June 28, 1970, to remember the anniversary of the Stonewall riots and those protests turned into Pride parades.

Online supporters of the group #NoJusticeNoPride compared the protest to such actions as the Stonewall Riots and ACT UP protests. But, no, I will not compare #NoJusticeNoPride to either. Stonewall and ACT UP were clear instances of a group of people fighting against institutions that criminalized us and left us to suffer and die. Stonewall happened because the community had been constantly harassed, jailed, and beaten by police. ACT UP started because people were dying of AIDS every day when there were little to no fucks given about those who were dying by the federal government and others. The Pride parade has not become such an institution.

Yes, the parade had corporate sponsors, but it also had community resources. Rerouting the parade meant there would be little to no attention given to the community resources that are there to help the trans and queer community or any other community for that matter. People who come to watch the parade sometimes learn about resources or organizations they did not know about. If I were a Latinx gay man or trans woman and did not speak or understand English, I would need to know where to go for resources. In the D.C. area, there are places that can help, like La Clinica del Pueblo, that provides resources to the LGBTQ Latinx community. Also, their mission is to is to create successful life stories among Transgender, Genderqueer and Gender Non-conforming, Gay, Lesbian and Bisexual people. So, by protesting, I feel #NoJusticeNoPride may have thwarted the individuals, especially young people, it claims to represent from being informed about the resources they need.

And information about resources is needed. According to statistics from the D.C. Department of Health among the 246 transgender persons diagnosed with HIV, 96.3 percent were linked to care, with fifty percent of them becoming linked to care within three months of diagnosis. Nearly three-quarters (72.8 percent) received any care in 2014, and, out of those, 68 percent were found to have received continuous care in 2014. Of all transgender persons diagnosed, 62.2 percent achieved viral suppression at last lab in 2014.

There are several ways of getting one's message across, but this form of protest may not be effective. However, I refuse to protest the protestors. Divisiveness among a minority only allows a majority to conquer them.

Just*in Time: September 2017

September 25, 2017

**Dear Justin,**

**I am very scared; I do not know who to talk to. I do not like using condoms, but I am on PrEP. So, I have protected myself from HIV. I know that I am open to being infected with other sexually transmitted diseases. I have tried to visit my primary care physician more often than just twice a year. However, I have developed a rash and it is getting worse. I visit my doctor next week, but I wanted to reach out to you to see what you think. I think I may have gotten syphilis because, in the Florida area where I live, syphilis infections have increased. Do you think this is because of PrEP [use without condoms]? I am thinking of going back to condoms because I have never had a sexually transmitted disease before.**
**—Fearful Florida Dude**

I hope all is well. Let me first thank you for writing in.

Let us start with your suspicion of a possible syphilis infection. Since you are on PrEP, doctors will require you to come in at least once every three months to make sure that, if you have been infected by a sexually transmitted infection (STI), it is caught early. The earlier a STI is detected the better, because it may prevent the development of other STIs, progression of the STI detected, and, in some cases, death. When PrEP is prescribed, physicians know that you are more susceptible to being infected with other STIs. I am not going to tell you that you have syphilis because that is your doctor's job, but I will tell you to see him or her as soon as you can.

Now I will go into some of the symptoms of syphilis and, yes, a rash is only one of the many skin symptoms. With a syphilis infection, you may experience ulcers, sores, and wart-like growths in your groin, and vaginal discharge. On your skin, you might experience ulcers, bumps, or rashes. Your body may experience weight loss, inflammation of the rectum, rashes on your palms and/or feet, fatigue, enlargement of lymph nodes, and a sore throat. Unlike some STIs, syphilis goes through stages of infection. The first stage is characterized by sores on the genitals, rectum, or mouth, which might go unnoticed because they are painless. When the sores heal a lot of people think they are in the clear, hence why there may be more syphilis infections than others. When the sores heal, the syphilis infection, if left untreated, will go into the second stage, which is the inevitable skin rash. This is the stage that most people notice that they may need to be checked by a physician. The third stage is the most severe and can damage many internal organs such as the eyes, nerves, brain, and the heart. So, since you are going to see your doctor next week, mention your symptoms and have your physician run a test for you.

Okay, I have to correct you and everyone who is reading this on something. We in the public health field are trying to get away from using the term "STD" as now we are trying to use the term "STI," because there is a difference. An STI is a broader and more encompassing description because some infections are curable and may not show any warning signs. If the infection changes a normal function of the human body, then it is considered a disease. It is more accurate to use the term STI and it is a reminder to the general population to get tested for possible infections because many infections have no symptoms.

Just an FYI for everyone: In 2015 Florida came out with its State Health Profile. According to the Centers for Disease Control and Prevention (2015) primary and secondary (P&S) syphilis (the stages in which syphilis is most infectious) remains one of Florida's main health issues, primarily among men who have sex with men (MSM). In Florida, the rate of primary and secondary syphilis was 6.6 per 100,000 in 2011 and 10.5 per 100,000 in 2015. Florida now ranks sixth in rates of P&S syphilis among fifty states. I have not been able to find the 2016 stats because I do not think they are out yet.

If you want to go back to using condoms that will be up to you. I cannot tell you how to protect yourself against STIs. But I will say I am a PrEP advocate and a condom advocate. Do what you feel is most comfortable for you. But do not be afraid. Weigh the possibilities and dangers. Empower yourself to take control of your own sexual health.


Just*in Time: October 2017: Staying Healthy in a Natural Disaster
October 11, 2017

In public health we know that when a natural disaster occurs it affects people living with chronic illnesses. HIV/AIDS itself is a disaster and compounding it with natural disasters like hurricanes will only hurt attempts at prevention, treatment, and livelihood. People need advice in times like these and I personally have been through a natural disaster that has affected me. There are things that people must keep in mind when dealing with a natural disaster, like the recent Hurricane Harvey, especially if they are infected with a chronic illness.

## Drink Only Potable Water

With almost every natural disaster water quality is directly affected. Water quality will decrease and may become unpotable (undrinkable). Consuming unpotable water will leave a person open to infections. If you are living with HIV, you may find yourself fighting off other infections. I suggest always keeping a supply of sealed water on hand. In my household, we stock gallons of water in case such an emergency occurs. We have been through storms where we must conserve water and those gallons of water truly did help.

## Medication Crunch Time

During a natural disaster it is imperative that people with chronic illnesses have their medication available to them. There is a chance that a person will lose medications or even run out, which will impede a person's treatment. There are ways that one may be able to work around this issue, such as contacting an organization that distributes unexpired medications. People who change medications may have some leftovers from their supply of unneeded medications and they may be able to donate the medication to persons affected by the natural disaster. I also suggest that you might want to keep a surplus of the medication you are on. I order a ninety-day supply of my HIV medication and order a new batch when I have only thirty days left of the medication. If you can afford it, I highly recommend this strategy.

## Do not Let Stigma Silence You

HIV stigma is still alive and well but to be treated and stay healthy you must be open and tell a healthcare provider about your condition if you have been moved to a new healthcare site. Tell them what medications you are on, when you last took your pills, and how many milligrams your medication is. You should have this all written down or documented somewhere in case you become separated from your medications.

## Be Wary of Sepsis

With flood waters rising it is crucial that people living with a chronic illness do not wade in water. You do not want to be cut or otherwise injured by sharp objects hiding beneath the surface. Becoming injured while in water leaves a person open to sepsis, which is a when a toxin-bearing bacterium infects the bloodstream and travels throughout the body. The risk of sepsis is increased with the elderly, and others with weakened immune systems. Infections that can lead to sepsis are pneumonia, kidney, and bloodstream, and/or stomach infections.

## Medical Records

Sometimes natural disasters can be predicted but often they will take you by surprise—or at least the effects of the disaster will. Remember that you will need your medical records and cards so that you can be administered care if and when the time comes. Many people keep their medical cards in their wallets or purses. I suggest making a copy of them and all other records to be put into a small safe that is water- and fireproof. Electronic records are also now available via apps.

I know that many of you in Houston and neighboring cities are suffering. I can only hope and pray that you are getting or will get the care you need. I also pray that you and your families are safe. There are people who are missing, hurt, and killed. I am asking not begging for all of you that are reading my column to reach out to those in the affected areas. By reaching out you never know how you can help. The smallest favor can be the biggest blessing. Shalom.

Just*in Time: HIV & Oral Health

November 22, 2017

Persons living with HIV must take extra care of their bodies and minds. I have this saying I repeat to myself when things do not go as well as I think they should go after a depressing doctor's appointment. "My body wasn't given the ability to fight off a virus constantly." This includes one's oral health; yes, I am talking about your teeth and gums, people. People may not know this but there are certain things of which people living with HIV need to stay conscious and cautious.

As several oral health issues can show up with people who are living with HIV, here are eight facts that one must know about HIV and the mouth. (Remember that, with any medical condition, you should consult a physician, preferably someone who specializes in HIV medicine.)

1. Problem: **Oral warts** (human papillomavirus, or HPV) can be transmitted sexually. Solution: The warts in your mouth can be frozen off or cut out.

2. Problem: **Dry mouth and tooth decay** can happen to anyone. Habits such as drinking coffee, alcohol, carbonated drinks, high sugar intake, and smoking cigarettes can give someone dry mouth and tooth decay.

Solution: Drink water! Water can help cleanse the mouth and body, prevent dry mouth, and cleanse your kidneys and liver; whose health is paramount when living with HIV.

3. Problem: **Candidiasis** (thrush) is basically a fungus or yeast that grows in your mouth. The symptoms are white lumps or red rashes inside your mouth. It is mostly found on the inside of your cheeks. Thrush can be very painful but there is hope.

Solution: Talk to your doctor about being prescribed anti-fungal medicines. Some medicine come in gel form. These medicines may ease your pain, but thrush will have to come out of your system on its own.

4. Problem: **Canker sores** (apthous ulcers) are open sores in your mouth and the back of your throat. They are usually caused by the types of food people eat, i.e., tomatoes, juices, or anything acidic, and spicy foods.

Solution: Some creams and gels work and, along with drinking water, should help soothe the pain.

5. Problem: **Cold sores** (herpes simplex type 1) happen to just about everyone, but with people infected with HIV the sores come back more often and more severe than in people who do not have HIV.

Solution: Antiviral drugs are available to manage the symptoms and reduce the longevity and intensity of the outbreaks.

6. Problem: **Gum disease** (gingivitis) is a major problem for people living with HIV. This condition causes pain and bleeding, and, if it goes unchecked by a dentist, then teeth will decay and fall out.

Solution: Brush your teeth daily. However, it is just as important to floss. When you first start this process, flossing might hurt, or your gums may bleed but it will subside in time. Try to floss every night before you go to bed. The number-one thing that is a turn off to any man/woman is bad breath.

7. Problem: **Kaposi's sarcoma** (KS), a type of cancer, can look like dark purple spots on the gums and on the back of the tongue.

Solution: When a HIV-positive person goes on antiretroviral therapy, the chance of having KS decreases exponentially.

8. Problem: **Shingles** (herpes zoster) can show up in the body as a painful rash, blisters, or lesions, which can show up on one side of the body, usually on the face, which includes the mouth, ears, pharynx (nasal or oral cavity), ears and larynx or torso area.

Solution: In 2006, the Food and Drug Administration (FDA) approved a vaccine called Zostavax. Zostavax is a live, attenuated vaccine that contains the same strain of virus. These conditions are all potentially very serious and you should see a dentist or doctor immediately to stay on top of your oral health. It is important! As you grow older with HIV, the virus could grow stronger. Preventative measures should be taken to ensure good healthy teeth and gums. Brush your teeth every day and try to floss before bed. I know that I sound like a toothpaste commercial, but oral health is a serious issue for everyone but especially people living with HIV.

Just*in Time: Language Matters

December 9, 2017

Language matters. It can promote prejudice and misinformation; it shapes our thinking about who and what has value in this world. Logging into a dating/hook-up app, like Grindr, is no excuse to log off of your brain or heart. Typos are excusable stigma is not!

So here are seven things that get the "thumbs down" emoji in these virtual communications.

**"I'm sorry."**

When someone says they are sorry I have HIV, I think, "Did we fuck or something?" Why are they sorry? Well, first think about it. They are sorry that you were infected, which is all well and good I suppose. But then take this opportunity to educate to say, "Don't be sorry for me, but be strong with me." A lot of people with this reaction are not really educated on what it means to live with HIV. Ask them if they know what the term "undetectable" means or what "PrEP" is. If they do not know, educate them.

**"You have HIV—thanks for telling me."**

Most online MSM dating apps, such as Grindr, come with an option in the profile to put what your HIV status is. So, if they ask me, it tells me that the other person did not read my profile and did not really care to. All they did was look at my picture and tried to hook up with me. I find that being upfront with my status also helps either facilitate discussion around sexual parameters, and/or it weeds out persons that I probably would not like to be sexual with or vice versa, which of course is fine by me.

"Are you trying to spread your disease, or something?"

The response (at least the one that I use) is, "No, I'm not." I would not wish the medical or doctor appointments and medication expenses on anyone. Having HIV is not easy; one can get used to the pills, appointments, and expenses but why would anyone want that? I myself am undetectable and many people do not know what undetectable is and do not know that the Centers for Disease Control and Prevention have themselves said that the risk of someone that has a sustained, undetectable viral load transmitting HIV is none. Also, there are several more STI besides HIV and I would not want to spread any of them. Plus, I would not want to risk my body to co-infection and then infect someone with two sexually transmitted infections at the same time, for example.

**"Your partner has HIV, too?"**

Now there is one thing about being open about your status online but another thing when someone asks about your partner's or spouse's HIV status. This is nobody's business. My response to this question would be to say, "This is really too personal to tell you and really it's his business to tell."

**"If you're partnered/married, why are you on here?"**

People are on social dating apps to hook up, date, or just to talk to others in the area to hopefully build a network of friends. But let us address this question. We have to understand that there are different types of relationships and not everyone practices monogamy. If you see someone is talking to you who is partnered/married and you do not agree with it, just say, "I'm not interested in hooking up with a partnered/married person" and move on. Also, on the flipside, the person who is partnered/married has to understand that some people are not interested in partnered/married people.

**"I'm not going on PrEP so sorry it's condoms or we are not fucking."**
Granted there are other STIs we all have to watch for, especially individuals on PrEP who do not use condoms, but we should support all who are empowered to protect themselves. We must consider that there will be individuals who will only strictly want to use condoms and individuals who do not and are on PrEP. I, for one, know there is a different feeling when having sex with and without a condom. But, besides that, we simply have to accept that some people only use PrEP, and some prefer condoms. My response to this would be, "Ohh okay well good luck" or "I could use condoms as well."

**"I can't hook up with you. I'm negative and I plan on staying that way."**
Whenever I encounter this attitude, I usually respond with saying, "I hope you do as well." I personally would never "spread" my virus to anyone. When you are upfront with your HIV status you may encounter this. Some people will refuse to have sex with you whether they are on PrEP or use condoms. But the response I have is used to support them in staying negative. You can also use this opportunity to educate them on HIV prophylaxis.

People will try to shame you because of your HIV status, but do not let them. Take the high road and do not go down the path of negativity. The more negative energy you put into your life, the more negative outputs you will have. Granted you can respond to any of the seven things any way you want—turning the other cheek, blocking, and not responding at all work just as well.

Just*in Time: Serodifferent Relationships & Resisting Stigma

by Justin B. Terry-Smith

January 26, 2018

Serodifferent relationships can work, but to be successful, partners (and those around them) need to be aware of how to empower themselves. Here are six issues to stay on top of in a relationship where at least one partner is HIV-positive, and one is HIV-negative. (I say "at least" and you know why—I support polyamory!)

**Do not slut-shame:** It is really important that in our HIV community we do not feel slut-shamed or slut-shame anyone else. All of us need support from our friends, family, and especially our partners. When that support is diminished, we, whether HIV-negative or positive, are more susceptible to depression and other dark energies. HIV-negative people should not be slut-shamed by others because they are on PrEP and they have the kind of sex they want to, and HIV-positive people should not be slut-shamed by those who stigmatize sex.

**Keep stress to a minimum:** Stress likes to creep into any relationship. The one thing about stress that not a lot of people know about is that it hurts the immune system. Whether you are positive or negative, nobody needs stress in their lives. A stressor may prompt someone into an action that benefits them, but this should be infrequent and not all the time.

**Safe/Safer sex:** There are many couples that are having this issue: The positive partner does not want to transmit the virus to his/her negative partner; nor does the negative partner want to acquire HIV. Both need to have a conversation about sexual practices. If the negative partner starts PrEP and wants to stop using condoms, yet the positive partner, even though on treatment and undetectable for a sustained period, and therefore unable to transmit HIV, still wants to use condoms—how do they move the relationship forward? Stay educated and engaged in evidence-based facts about HIV. Without this knowledge and without communicating with your partner, fear might persist. And fear feeds stigma. Everyone has to make their own choice in their own health to take empowerment into their own hands. But do not be scared to be empowered; be scared of the fear stigma breeds…no pun intended.

**Resentment sucks:** We as HIV-positive people have to take a little better care of ourselves than most. Remember our human bodies were not meant to fight a virus for years on end. Taking pills, going to the doctor at least three times a year, making sure your T-cell counts are high and you remain undetectable can definitely have its range of emotions. Having a partner who does not have to make those decision or go through the challenges can be tough. But we must remember not to resent them for that. They are people just like we are, and we must understand that they are going through pain as well. Having a partner who is HIV positive can be hurtful, too, but we must understand that it is not a picnic in the park, and we have to be patient because we would want someone to be there for us too.

**Children:** Children are simple: You either want children or you do not. If a serodifferent male-male couple seeks a surrogate, there is still the challenge of who is going to be the "donor." Technology has made leaps and bounds and now either one can be the genetic parent, thanks to sperm cleansing. Sperm cleansing allows doctors to separate the infected seminal fluid from the semen cells, which are then inserted into one or many eggs to produce children. According to the International Assisted Reproduction Center HIV-positive sperm donation has zero risk for surrogate mothers. Also, if an HIV-positive female wants to carry a child the pregnant woman must be on ART every day and stay healthy throughout pregnancy in order to not transmit HIV to the child. To further prevent infection after the child is born, the child is given ART right away for four to six weeks.

**Death—that's life:** Death comes for us all and we cannot be afraid of it. Back in the first decades of the epidemic, there were people who were infected with HIV and had only years, sometimes months, to live. Now the treatment for those living with HIV exists and is getting better all the time. Those who are on treatment for HIV have been known to live just as long as people who are HIV-negative. So, if you are negative and your main concern is that you will outlive your positive partner, think again. People also need to understand that just because you are positive you should not go through the remainder of your life with the fear of dying. People walk out of their houses and get hit by cars, have heart attacks, brain aneurysms, and die. Do not let HIV dictate your life, whether you are positive or negative!

Just*in Time: 7 Reasons Why We Still Fight

February 26, 2018

Put simply: It is Not Over. And we are not ready to put AIDS activism in a museum! Here are seven reasons why HIV/AIDS activism is still important.

## 1. HIV is not a thing of the past

People think HIV is a problem of the eighties and nineties, but it is still an ongoing public health issue. And it has been going on for longer that you might think. Did you know HIV first reared its ugly fucking face in the United States in the late 1960s? A teenager from Missouri named Robert Rayford died from pneumonia, but at the time doctors were very puzzled about his other symptoms as well. After much debate in 1988, an autopsy found the presence of HIV antibodies and lesions from Kaposi's sarcoma. Rayford has been described as the earliest case of HIV/AIDS in North America having been infected with a virus closely related or identical to HIV. How can we let a disease that has been around that long in the United States still manage to kill Americans?

## 2. New generations can become complacent

I remember how AIDS-related conditions would kill people less than a year after a person had been diagnosed. This was truly sad, and many people had to live through watching their friends die, attending a funeral of a fallen friend a couple times a week, and/or being a caretaker for someone dying of one or more opportunistic infections. We should understand that we can and should never forget our past and how HIV has impacted us. The more we remember our past, the more of a chance that we will not repeat it.

## 3. There is still no cure

In the early days, a cure was promised. It did not come. The promises stopped. Now researchers are still dedicated to finding preventative and therapeutic vaccines, but they are more careful about reporting on their progress.

## 4. Every little bit counts

In the federal budget there is never enough money for HIV. If we want to end this epidemic, we need to raise the funds. Never sit down and complain about something—get off your ass and do something. Even on Facebook you can start a virtual fundraiser and have proceeds go to a HIV/AIDS organization that might even be giving services to a person you know.

## 5. Stigma is still alive and well

We can decrease HIV stigma by educating the general population. But stigma will always be around until there is a cure. I see it day in and day out. People do not want to be friends with others because of HIV or date them or even take the time to listen to them. This is appalling, and it needs to stop. And, as an ally, it starts or stops with you. You are the one that either can be an asshole or a good friend.

## 6. Firing of HIV advisory officials

With certain leaders firing or removing HIV professionals from their posts, there needs to be a more activism. The more and more leaders we have in our fight, the more social change can occur. It will not occur in a hurry, but it will cause the start of a discussion. These discussions may seem monotonous, but, if someone is listening, that starts the spark to fuel the fire.

## 7. Underserved communities

Do you actually think that everyone has the same opportunities to have access to medical treatment in this country? Think again. According to the Health and Human Services (HHS), despite improvements, differences persist in healthcare quality among racial and ethnic minority groups. Also, people in low-income families also experience poorer quality care. Just an FYI: Disparities in quality of care are common. For example, adults aged sixty-five and over received worse care than adults aged eighteen to forty-four for thirty-nine percent of quality measures. African Americans received worse care than Whites for forty-one percent of quality measures. Latinx/Hispanics received worse care than non-Hispanic Whites for thirty-nine percent of measures. Asian/Pacific Islanders and American Indian/Alaskan Natives received worse care than Whites for nearly thirty percent of quality measures. Poor people received worse care than high-income people for forty-seven percent of measures. The more disparities we have with our care, the more illnesses and deaths will occur. The end game is to Get to Zero!

Just*in Time: Staying Healthy When Living with HIV
March 23, 2018

My field is public health, and we look at the big picture quite often. But really public health also means you. We can make changes as individuals to improve our health, so here are some of the important strategies to stay healthy when living with HIV.

### Exercise, gym, or no gym

Yes, I know that, at the beginning of the year, many of us (me included) make New Year's resolutions and then it is March, and no progress has been made. Mine was to get to the gym, the same gym for which I have a membership but never use. Exercise, however, is one resolution I intend to keep. In terms of living with HIV, exercising can help those of us who have experienced weight loss by increasing body mass. We may also suffer from increased levels of blood sugars and fats, such as cholesterol, which can increase the risk of some serious long-term health issues. Exercise reduces the risk of many of these issues, such as Type 2 diabetes and osteoporosis.

### Eat healthy

For my own personal spiritual reasons, I have cut pork out of my diet. Of course, I am not telling you to cut pork out of your diet. We all have to do what makes us happy....OINK. HIV is a tricky fucker, and it likes to dictate when we are hungry or should not eat. A lot of people do not eat three times a day, but it is important that persons with HIV eat three healthy meals a day.

Fruits and vegetables give the body antioxidants, and antioxidants help protect your immune system.

Carbs! Now before you say, "Hell no," hear me out. Carbohydrates actually give your body energy—it is like gassing up your car. Also make sure you get fiber in your diet as it helps fight against lipodystrophy or wasting.

Change to sea salt—that is what the Internet seems to be telling us. Okay, maybe changing to sea salt is not the best advice but do decrease your salt and sugar intake. Too much in one's diet can increase one's chances of heart disease. People living with HIV are already at an increased chance of getting heart disease.

People who are living with HIV need more protein in their diet, as it helps restore, repair, and preserve all the cells in the body, maintains hormone levels, and enzymes.

Many ASOs provide nutritional services to help guide your diet, or even provide necessary food missing from your pantry.

**More pills?!**
Some vitamins and minerals, such as zinc, iron, selenium, and vitamin B12, may not be well absorbed in people with HIV. I suggest if you cannot find these in foods you like, there are pills that contain vitamins and minerals that your body may need. Yes, I know. Who in the hell would want to take more pills? Well, if you do not, you do not, but you should at least consider the option. I personally take vitamin D pills daily and glucosamine as well.

**Mental health**
If you have HIV, it is important to take care of both your physical and mental health. When you are living with HIV you have an increased chance of mental health conditions than persons who are HIV-negative. According to the National Institute of Mental Health (NIMH), in 2015, about

eighteen percent of American adults in the United States had a mental illness, and this can include mental conditions such as stress, depression and anxiety. Resources may be in place around you. Sometimes it is best to be around people who are going through what you are, and who understand your challenges. People living with HIV often join a support group, meeting others in a safe and supportive environment. HIV support groups exist in major cities, but what if you live somewhere without support? There are supportive phone apps that can put you in touch with someone to talk to.

**Meditate**

I do not mean to sound too New Agey, but meditation works for me. When I get stressed out, I get on my knees (stop thinking about that!) and close my eyes. I let all the stress, negative energy, and thoughts go, with every breath. For me, it helps decrease depression, anxiety, and stress. According to the National Center for Complementary and Integrative Health (NCCIH) (2017), meditation also decreases blood pressure, symptoms of irritable bowel syndrome, and insomnia, and increases calmness and physical relaxation, improving psychological balance, coping with illness, and enhancing overall health and well-being.

Just*in Time: Meth Use & HIV
April 24, 2018

Do you ParTy? I get this question all the time on apps like Grindr, Jack'd, Scruff or Growlr. Okay, more on Grindr. But I have the same reply no matter what app the person hits me up on, "I'm not interested." Do not get me wrong, back in my twenties, Papa was a rolling stoned, young man.

Now I am thirty-eight and I am a little wiser and a less of a wild child. But I can say I have never ever tried meth and I have no intention to in the future. I can honestly say I do not judge anyone who does meth, but I cannot give any part of myself to them. It is not judgment, but I cannot trust the person on it. Being HIV-positive, I can only imagine how it interacts with one's body. Instead of complaining about it, I have decided to educate myself and others on the detriments of meth to your HIV-positive body.

So, let us first look at some basic information about meth. Meth is a shorter name for crystal methamphetamine (CM), also known as crystal meth. Meth is a highly addictive drug that is considered a stimulant. Meth can be injected, snorted, smoked, and/or swallowed. A lot of people insert it into their rectums as well. Meth is very inexpensive and can last as long as two days. For example, I knew of a man who drove high all the way from Atlanta to Washington, D.C., just because he wanted to meet a guy have sex and get more Meth.

• **Errors in judgment.** Like a lot of drugs, meth lowers one's inhibitions and ability to make sound decisions by impairing one's judgment. When you are high on meth, you are more likely to engage in riskier sex.

• **Dick soft?** If you are a person with a penis, sometimes meth use is a cause of making your dick soft. Yeah, I said it. This can lead to people using erectile dysfunction medication on top of meth to stay hard. Your body might become dependent on the drug and the Viagra to stay hard for a longer period of time.

• **Bottoms up!** Many people engage in bottoming when on crystal meth because they claim it feels better and they can take a bigger dick. Well, the ugly truth is that meth increases the risk for tissue tears in your ass because it causes mucosal dryness.

• **Sharing is not caring.** When injecting meth, you do run the risk of transmitting HIV or other STIs like hepatitis C.

• **Hungry, bitch?!** Meth reduces your appetite and weight. When you are HIV-positive it is important for you to eat. One, because it helps sustain nutrients in the body; two, your immune system needs fuel to fight off other infections; and three, if you are on an anti-HIV treatment regimen, then you need to eat a certain number of calories with your HIV medication for it to be properly absorbed by your body.

• **Depression.** Many people do drugs on a regular basis to try to get away from feelings of depression and isolation. When someone is on meth, they are not thinking about what in their life is causing their depression or isolation. After a binge of being high for days on end, the user is often faced with a pummeling by those same feelings.

• **Internal effects.** Meth gives you a high chance of a stroke or heart attack, because of its effects on the heart. Meth increases your heart rate, blood pressure, and body temperature.

• **HIV into AIDS.** Meth use accelerates HIV progression into an AIDS diagnosis. The National AIDS Treatment Advocacy Project revealed the outcomes of a controlled study from the University of California, San Diego, that discovered an unswerving connection between meth and T-cell activation and proliferation in HIV-positive men. The study participants who did use the drug in the study showed a higher risk of cognitive impairment and a faster development into AIDS-defining illnesses.

Meth is a big problem in our community. But there are resources that can help you. In just about every major city there are rehabs/drug addiction treatment centers, and, if you do not want to do that, then there are many support groups that focus on meth addiction. It is up to you if you want help or not. I am nobody's judge, and I am in no way trying to tell anyone how to live. Just know that if you engage in this activity, there are consequences. Your body is already fighting HIV, you do not want it fighting against meth as well.

Just*in Time: Life Is Not Over
June 27, 2018

I find that a lot of newly diagnosed people living with HIV believe that their life is over. I said it before that, when I found out that I was positive, I first thought: What are my parents going to think? My second thought was: What am I to do now I cannot have any biological children of my own? My third thought was that I am going to die. Then I thought: What was the point of even going back to school?
Looking back at all of these statements and questions, I think to myself that all of them have either been misinformed or have been answered favorably. Presently, my parents are very proud of me and love the work that I do; HIV-positive persons can have children without the child acquiring HIV or they can adopt as well. And I do not plan on dying anytime soon. The education piece was much harder to think about.

Thinking about how education has fulfilled my life thus far it only felt natural to go back to school, until I became HIV-positive. I had fulfilled at least one year of college education before I became positive. It took a while to get back to school, but I did. I went back, and I went back on a mission.

I earned my associate's in Communications from Axia College and, in 2009, I went on to earn my bachelor's in Political Science. I did not want to stop because, as I excelled in my education, my job prospects went up and I was able to earn more money. This allowed me to eventually get off of Maryland AIDS Drug Assistance Program (MADAP). Just in case you did not know, MADAP ensures that people living with HIV/AIDS in Maryland have access to the medication they need to stay healthy and is a statewide program and is funded primarily through the Ryan White CARE Act. MADAP pays for medications for eligible clients with no insurance and helps clients with insurance by paying for eligible co-pay and deductible costs so they can get their medication.

In 2015 I received my Master's degree in Public Health (MPH), a field that I am passionate about. A month after I received my MPH, I was interviewed and hired in the public health arena for my 9-to-5 job; my activism has been in HIV since 2003. In my heart I knew I was a public health advocate, and that education would further solidify my expertise in the field. This year I was awarded my Doctorate in Public Health and now I feel more fulfilled than ever. How I am going to use my doctorate? I do not know yet, but what I do know is that I shall use it wisely. I am not telling you to go out and get a doctorate, but what I am saying is that all ambitions and dreams do not end with HIV.

People often forget their dreams or put them on the back burner because of HIV, but this cannot be. Fulfill your potential; use this experience to help others going through the same thing to fulfill their own potential. Use opportunities like this one to further educating others on HIV.

What some people do not understand is that sometimes life is not straightforward for some of us. As the road curves, we then use our life experiences to dictate what we will do professionally in life or what we feel passionate about. I know for my life it is both—straight lines and curves. Before I became HIV-positive, for example, I already knew and had dated people who were positive. I actually started working at an HIV non-profit in 2003. I watched friends die and suffer because of HIV and I knew I had to do something. I knew that I could not turn my head or idly watch as my friends became affected by being infected with HIV. A lot of my friends became complacent with being positive; they died either because they were not educated enough to get resources, or they thought because they were HIV-positive they could just easily take pills at any time and be okay and they would often die because of not taking their meds until it was too late. I knew I needed to make resources available to my community so that another friend did not die in vain. So, I fulfilled one of my dreams of having an education. I know they are proud of what I have accomplished, and I will continue to make them proud by fulfilling more of my dreams.

Sleep well and have pleasant dreams, everyone!


Just*in Time: HIV & the Military
July 23, 2018

Since I am a veteran of the military (a disabled Air Force vet) there are several dates throughout the year that touch me: Memorial Day, to remember all who have fallen in the line of duty, Veterans Day. to remember all of us who have served in the military, and then there is the Fourth of July, when we remember how the United States of American was able to fight off the British to gain its independence. I also remember all those who are currently serving.
Often, I come across people who are unclear about what happens or what might happen to someone who becomes HIV-positive while in the military. Let me set the facts straight and also give you my take about military policy.

**HIV-positive=No Admittance to the military:** Section 5-3-a states: "Applicants for accession who have no military status of any kind at the time of testing and who are confirmed HIV infected will not be enlisted or appointed in any component of the Army."

Even though we presently know that Undetectable = Untransmittable, people still live-in fear of acquiring HIV. But also, the concern could be that there will be someone who does not take their own medications to stay undetectable and might transmit the virus. Sex, however, is a two-way and sometimes three-way street. We are all responsible for our own sex lives.

**HIV-positive=Not Deployable:** Many of us who join the military have dreams of being deployed to other countries. Some of us also long to go to a hot spot where there is combat in order to fight for our country. When you, as a member of the military, are diagnosed as HIV-positive, that will not happen. Again, even though we know that those living with HIV can take care of themselves and respond to meds to the point of viral suppression, policy is still driven by fear. Positive soldiers will not be deployed or assigned overseas, nor will they be permitted to perform official duties overseas for any duration of time. Soldiers confirmed to be HIV-positive while stationed overseas will be reassigned to the United States. Some policy is changing; according to StarsandStripes.com, the Navy allows HIV-positive sailors and Marines to be placed at some military installations outside of the United States, and on certain large ships.

**PrEP=Positive Change:** Since the FDA approval of pre-exposure prophylaxis (PrEP), and its availability in healthcare settings, there has been a more sex-positive attitude among those educated about HIV prevention and harm reduction. PrEP is available to military personnel, but not without difficulty. In general, the prevention option paves the way for there to be less stigma for military personnel who are diagnosed with HIV.

**Different Perspectives on HIV Prevention:** The Navy allows its personnel to take PrEP. According to Military.com, Air Force military personnel, however, have been denied PrEP, with officials citing safety concerns. The Air Force requires a waiver for its pilots on flying status to have a prescription for PrEP. Yet, according to reports, no Air Force waivers have been created since PrEP's approval in 2012.

**Money=Power:** According to Military.com, the Air Force invests between $3 to $12 million into each pilot over the course of his or her career; now add HIV medications to that. The military may not be willing to put up the money to pay for HIV preventative measure such as PrEP, let alone anti-HIV regimens.

As a disabled 9/11 veteran who is HIV positive, I feel the military has done a major disservice to those who have acquired HIV while serving in the military and those of us who are already positive and want to join the military. Individuals living with HIV and engaged in care have the right to serve and fight for their country. Regulations that prevent HIV prophylaxis from being accessible to any military personnel is a disgrace. One can only hope that the military will do better in treating its personnel better—with compassion and goodness.

## Just*in Time: Navigating the HIV Closet

Just*in Time

by Justin B. Terry-Smith

August 29, 2018

What do you do when feeling rejected by family members when you come out of the HIV closet?
I thought about the month of August and how it is a big month for my family.

My father's and mother's birthdays are both in August, and, to celebrate those two dates, I always send them a little something in the mail. My father will tell me and my brother to only call or send him a card. I will usually send my mother her favorite flowers. Also, my brother's wedding anniversary is in August as well. He had an awesome wedding in Jamaica and married a beautiful woman that I am proud to call sister. August is also when I said "I do" to the most wonderful man in the world. So, when I think of August, I think of my family, but not all of us are lucky enough to have a supportive family.

Coming out of the HIV closet is even harder without support of one's family. Here are six points to remember as you consider having and/or navigating this discussion:

**Reactions from family members**
You are going to get a whole spectrum of reactions. Some are going to be supportive and others will hurt you to your core. Keep the mindset that the family members that shun you are the ones with the problem. There is nothing wrong with you.

**Searching out supportive family**
You will need the strength of the supportive family members. Even though they are not infected

themselves and will not know your struggle, you will still need someone in your family that is supportive and that will show you acceptance and love. Try not to lash out at them.

**Put that negative energy elsewhere**

The frustration of not being accepted by one's family can tear you up inside. I understand. However, aggressive behavior on your part may come out in ways that are sometimes not healthy for others. Time to turn that energy into positive energy. Some examples include going to the gym, writing your feelings out on paper, going to the spa, etc.

**Families can be chosen**

This is especially true in the LGBTQ community, and there is strength in numbers. When your established family rejects you, you need to find a network and quickly. In a network of individuals living with HIV, there is a family and support. You will have a network to share similar stories, to find out what to do in case a specific problem arises and help each other through thick and thin. Now that sounds like family to me.

**Educate, educate, educate**

My family members asked me a lot of questions when they found out I am HIV-positive. You have to keep in your mind that they might not know anything about being HIV-positive and their questions may seem insulting. For example, one of my family members asked, "How long did the doctor give you?" That was over thirteen years ago. Obviously, nobody knows when their last day on earth will be. But I did not lose my cool; instead, I explained that not even he knows how long he has on this earth.

**Do not let stigma in**

Some of your family members might view you as "dirty" when you tell them you are HIV-positive. I had a family member tell me she was surprised that I was dating. She even went as far as to tell me, "Be careful because that's how you got in trouble in the first place." I thought to myself how insensitive she was being. I talked to her about how it hurt me to hear her say that because it perpetuates stigma.

Sometimes your family means well, and they have no idea the detriment that they do. Over time sometimes family will apologize for their ignorance, as long as they understand what they have done. The worst part about this is sometimes it is too late to be regretful. We all need to understand that education is the key.


Just*in Time: Know Your Healthcare Worker

October 10, 2018

Hey, everyone, I hope all is well. Fall is here and the first holiday that comes to mind is Labor Day. Does anyone know what this holiday is about? And, no, it is not about pregnant women going into labor. Labor Day is more about the labor movement and the contributions that workers have made to the strength, prosperity, laws, and well-being of the country. This month, I would like to shine a spotlight on those who work with us to keep us healthy. I know there are a lot of us that absolutely hate having to deal with doctors or any public health professional, but maybe knowing more about what public health professionals do and why they can be an important part of our HIV journey might take the sting out.

**Case Manager**

Many of us who are newly diagnosed are assigned a case manager to help with accessing medication and other resources. One of the biggest complaints that patients have with their case managers is that they are unresponsive to needs. I am not giving excuses, but I am going to give another perspective. Case managers who work in the HIV community often have too much of a caseload, especially if they are in an urban setting. They see people day in and day out, all day long. The case managers will not know you by name sometimes and often will not remember you. A solution is to get to know your case manager as they will be a lifeline to you. They might already know but let them know your vulnerabilities and talk to them on a regular basis so that they have a more interpersonal relationship with you.


**Internal Medicine/Primary Care Doctor**

One of the first things I did was seek out a doctor for myself. Since being diagnosed with HIV in 2006 I have seen four doctors. I finally found one who is an excellent physician. Dr. A. in NW D.C. is amazing. Before Dr. A., I had three other doctors who I felt treated me like a number. There was no personality when it came to the visits and it was often hard to get in contact with them when I had a question. When I finally switched to Dr. Ang, I felt like he actually cared about me as a person and not just because I had HIV. He has a great system in place. I see him every three months and, on every visit, I have a blood and urine test. I like thorough doctors and I like that he knows me and my family. If you are going to a doctor and you feel like just a number, it is time to get a new doctor.

## Dentist

Dentists work too hard to protect the general community by instilling knowledge in us about how to follow a good oral hygiene regimen. Many people hate going to the dentist and often complain about how they are frightened to go. But we have to go because we need to prevent gingivitis, halitosis, and other infections and conditions of the mouth. Lots of people complain that dentists who are not in private practice do not have the experience or knowledge to do good work. Honestly, please keep in mind, they are working with what they have. Many dentists make a salary as low as 30K a year. They also work on patients who have neglected their oral hygiene for years and sometimes only because they are on the lower end of the socioeconomic spectrum. A lack of dental insurance coverage is a travesty in this country and that is also another reason why people cannot get to a dentist right away or at all. But do not blame the dentist; blame the system.

## Pharmacist

Now the main concern that I hear from people is that they are not getting their prescriptions filled on time. I have seen people call their pharmacist and curse them out because they have not received their medications when expected. There are many reasons to consider when expecting your pharmacist to have your medications ready or mailed to you in a timely manner. Call your doctor first to check to see if they have sent in your prescription to your pharmacist. Understand the pharmacist cannot do anything until your doctor sends in the prescription. Another word of advice is to order the prescription early; in case something goes wrong you will have enough time to alleviate the problem and still stay compliant with your medication. They have a lot of patients that they work hard for and with, so do not think you are the only one on their list.

I chose to focus on these four public health professionals because I have the most experience with them. I have gone to see all four types of professionals named above when I was uninsured, underinsured, and fully insured. I have felt agitated and frustrated with all four, but now I understand what they go through day in and day out. But of course, living with HIV is not easy either. We all have to work together and fight the good fight.

Just*in Time: Destigmatizing Sex Work

Just*in Time

by Justin B. Terry-Smith

November 4, 2018

Happy Halloween, everyone. This month I will be addressing stigma and sex workers. Sex workers can be of all genders, sexual orientations, races, and any sex. They face so many challenges created by people's negative opinions of their professions, HIV stigma, police brutality, etc. We need to address these issues in our community as a whole to decrease discrimination, stigma, and HIV acquisitions.

According to the CDC (2016), sex workers are "people who exchange sex for money or nonmonetary items" and are at increased risk of acquiring or transmitting HIV and other STIs because they are more likely to engage in risky sexual practices and substance use.

So, what are some factors that keep sex workers at risk for acquiring HIV/STIs?

**Police Brutality**

In a 2008 report, "Move Along: Policing Sex Work in Washington, D.C.," by the Alliance for a Safe & Diverse DC, thirty-eight percent of the participants in the survey reported abuse (both verbal and physical) from police. Seventy-five percent of transgender and 82.4 percent of Latinx sex workers reported that their treatment while in jail was worse than others that were in jail with them. How can sex workers rely on help from the police when they are constantly being abused by the very ones who are supposed to be protecting them? Also, after being abused by police, 8.6 percent of the survey participants said that the police took or destroyed their safer sex supplies.

**Discrimination**

People often discriminate against sex workers because of the negative perception that sex workers are disposable. This is not true. We have to start looking at sex workers as members of our society who deserve the right to be known and counted. Consider supporting organizations that advocate for sex workers, especially those run by sex workers.

## Access to PrEP

Pre-exposure prophylaxis (PrEP) is an opportunity for sex workers to protect themselves against HIV infection. Luckily, according to the Global Advocacy for HIV Prevention, the drug Truvada, which is the medication used in the only PrEP regimen currently in use, is available through most private insurance and Medicaid. Gilead Sciences, which makes Truvada, also has two programs that can help you pay for PrEP (Medication Assistance Program and Gilead Advancing Access program). But how can someone pay for or even have access to PrEP when their very livelihood is constantly being attacked and there is no information available to properly advise sex workers of the benefits of this relatively new prevention tool? We must do more to ensure access to PrEP (and PEP).

## Male Sex Workers

As we know, men who have sex with men (MSM) are in one of the highest risk demographics to acquire HIV. In a 2015 study by Amanja Verhaegh-Haasnoot et al., in a group of 212 male participants who identified as male sex workers, forty percent tested positive for HIV/STIs. Fourteen percent of the 801 female sex workers who participated in the same study also tested positive for HIV/STIs. Male sex workers also reported having fewer clients in the same study. Knowing this fact, it is very possible that fewer clients means the male sex workers were more apt to have raw sex because the client will give them more money.

Sex work is one of the oldest professions in our nation, and luckily technology has allowed sex work to go mainstream and, in some ways, legally. It is not up to us to judge anyone for the work they do. The more judgment you give, the more you should feel ashamed…not them.

Just*in Time: On Circumcision

Just*in Time

by Justin B. Terry-Smith

January 22, 2019

During the holidays I am sure many of us had a Christmas tree, Hanukkah bush or Solstice scrub. But my question is, did you trim it or leave it untrimmed?

The controversy of wanting or having your penis circumcised has gone on for generations and will continue to happen. I have had boyfriends in my past that were cut and uncut, and personally I have no problem with either. I am cut myself and since I do not remember being circumcised as a baby, I really do not have a problem with myself being cut. Also, we must remember that in certain religions and spiritualities it is thought that a circumcision of a man's penis is his covenant with G-d. There have been several anti-circumcision movements of men that are upset about their own circumcisions because they did not consent to having the procedure performed; also, anti-circumcision activists cite that circumcision is painful and risky for babies. Fun fact: A 2012 Vice article states, "The U.S. circumcision rate (meaning how many newborns undergo the procedure) is officially placed at around 56%, which is lower than it once was but still far higher than other parts of the world. One-fourth of the planet's men are Muslim, and many are circumcised for religious reasons, as are most Jews, but the majority of European, Asian, and Central and South American countries don't practice ritual foreskin removal, and the World Health Organization estimates only 30% of all men are circumcised." In 2007 the World Health Organization advised heterosexual African males to get circumcisions in order to prevent against the transmission of HIV. Honestly, when I first heard that, it did not make any sense to me whatsoever. But it had me wondering, what are the public health positives and negatives of male circumcision?

**Positive Effects**

• Circumcision protects heterosexual men, by reducing HIV transmission by sixty percent

• Circumcision protects homosexual men, by reducing HIV transmission by fourteen percent

• Circumcision has been suggested for older boys and men to treat phimosis (the inability to retract foreskin), balanitis (inflammation), paraphimosis (inability of the foreskin to return to its original location), and/or infections.

• Easier hygiene

• Decreased risk of penile cancer and urinary tract infections

**Negative Effects**

• Some risks include bleeding, permanent injury, inflammation, and pain.

• Loss of nerve endings and nerve damage

• Keratinization, which is when a circumcision exposes a normally covered part of the skin which can cause glans to become abnormally dried out and thickened

- Premature ejaculation
- Decreased sexual pleasure and lower orgasm intensity

Circumcision continues to be a source of contention for some people. Many countries, especially in Europe, have tried to ban male circumcision. Iceland is slated to become the first European country to ban circumcision. This has sparked controversy in two main communities, especially. Iceland's population of about 336,000 which includes very small Jewish and Muslim communities. It is estimated that about 250 Jews and about 1,500 Muslims live in the country. Circumcision in both religions is widespread. Circumcision is considered a sign of belonging to the wider Islamic community and a form of cleanliness. In Judaism circumcision is considered a covenant with G_d.

In the United States there has been no legislature on the books to ban circumcision. There was an attempt in San Francisco seven years ago to ban circumcision; however, in October 2011 California passed a law protecting circumcision from local efforts to ban circumcisions. Each state has its own laws focused on circumcision and are asked to sometimes intervene when the parents cannot come to a decision on whether or not to circumcise their son. The United States will probably have a tougher time at banning circumcision because foreskin removal is common practice throughout the country and also some people say the benefits far outweigh the risks.

I can see both sides of this argument, but as a Doctor of Public Health I have to think about safety and long-term effects. Both are considered when coming to this decision. This writer, as of right now, is in favor of circumcision but only because of the medical benefits.

We all have our personal preference but what happens when personal preferences get in the way of religious rites? Whether or not you are cut or uncut, you need to know and be informed of the pros and the cons of circumcision. As for my personal preference…a dick is still a dick.


Just*in Time: Dating Sites & Living with HIV
February 13, 2019

So, here we are again. It is time for that commercialized holiday we call Valentine's Day, or Lover's Day for those of us who do not like St. Valentine. Being infected with HIV can be rough if you are looking for a little romance, but what can be rougher is being rejected because of it. Personally, I can say I was lucky to find my soulmate and husband but not many of us are that lucky. Many of us have now decided that we will only date other people living with HIV. I asked a couple of people why they would only date HIV-positive people and I heard people say that they like the fact that the person they are dating knows what they are going through, that they like not using a condom and that they feel more supported; all these factors were quite interesting to me. When I was dating, it was hard to disclose, but I did eventually. As I became more comfortable with my HIV status, it became easier and easier to disclose to my partners. Also, now that PrEP and U=U have come into play should we as HIV-positive people only date other HIV-positive people?

I did a little bit more research and looked into HIV dating sites. Of course, a lot of them catered to both HIV-positive and negative singles. There were many choices and most had the typical dating questions for singles like, do you plan on getting married? Do you want kids? What are you looking for in your partner? But also, they had questions on whether or not those looking for love were undetectable or on PrEP.

I have dated HIV-negative and positive men before and to me there was no difference. When I have been rejected because of my HIV status I have learned to say in my own head, "FUCK YOU….NEXT!!" Honestly, if you cannot say that chances are you are going to beat yourself up or at least, to a small degree, feel badly because of the rejection. Just say, "FUCK YOU" and keep it moving. Why waste your time feeling bad about something you have no control over? Ignorance is bliss and now you should let them go in peace.

I started thinking about HIV-positive singles sites again and I asked myself, "Are they really necessary? And, if so, can someone tell me why?"

In my opinion my answer is, Yes, they are necessary. One of the main reasons why I would think that positive dating sites are necessary is that people are tired of rejection. I know plenty of people that go through anxiety just by going on a date and having to think about how they are going to disclose their HIV status to someone who is negative. Then you have to think about how stigma affects a person. People do not want to be looked down upon because of their HIV status.

So, they feel that they have no pressure about disclosing if they go on a positive dating website. There is no added pressure of lying or disclosing one's status just to find love.

Another question arose from my research: Why should HIV-positive people have to feel as though they have to go to these dating websites to feel a certain level or acceptance? My answer is we should not have to. There is too much education on HIV out there for ignorant people to reject you because of your HIV status. It is wrong. But we all have our "preferences," don't we? Again, let us not agonize over ignorant people who obviously only see the virus rather than seeing you for the beautiful person you are. You can only be who you are.

Trust me, someone is going to love you regardless of your HIV status. I did not think I would find love, but I will have been married for ten years in August and we have been together for about thirteen years. In those thirteen years we have adopted two beautiful sons (now twenty-two and twenty-0ne years old), my husband supported me while getting my doctorate and we continue on this journey together. It has been and will continue to be an adventure.

And status had nothing to do with it!


Just*in Time: Testicular Cancer Prevention
April 19, 2019

Just*in Time
by Justin B. Terry-Smith

Here we are in April, the month where a lot of us think about Easter and Easter egg hunts. As adult men, I am suggesting that those of us with testicles go on our own "egg hunt"! Why? Testicular cancer is serious business and checking one's own "eggs" is paramount to staying healthy.

I started thinking about HIV-positive singles sites again and I asked myself, "Are they really necessary? And, if so, can someone tell me why?" Testicular cancer can affect all men, no matter our serostatus. There is very little evidence that having HIV is a factor in having an increased risk of testicular cancer, but it is important that, as a public health issue we must be informed of how to protect ourselves and what to look for.

According to the American Cancer Society there are different types of testicular cancers, but doctors can analyze the cells of the cancer to see what type of cancer it is and figure out what treatment is best.

Typically, cancer cells of the testicles are known as germ cells. The germ cells are made up of two types of tumors called seminomas and non-seminomas. The Cancer Center states that seminomas and non-seminomas are very different.

The seminoma tumors are categorized into two types of tumors. The classical seminoma usually occurs in men between the ages of thirty and fifty. The spermatocytic seminomas are usually found in men around or over the age of fifty-five. Even though both types of seminoma tumors are found in all ages, the classical seminoma is more commonly found.

The non-seminoma is categorized into four types. These types of tumors are usually found in teenagers and people in their early forties. The tumors are embryonal carcinoma, yolk sac carcinoma, choriocarcinoma, and teratoma. Embryonal carcinoma cells grow very fast and can quickly spread outside of the testicles. Yolk sac carcinoma cells are shaped like yolks and are very common, especially in children or young adults. Yolk sac carcinoma usually responds very well to chemotherapy. Teratoma cancer cells look like a three-layered embryo under a microscope.

Okay, now that we have the technical stuff out of the way, let us talk about prevention and treatment.

Drop Those Eggs: Many men are born with undescended testicles, that is, testicles that have not moved into their proper position. Having undescended testicles increases your risk for testicular cancer. This condition is easily rectified with surgery and usually is detected at birth.

Feel Those Eggs: Yes, men, feel those testicles. It is time for a self-exam. The American Cancer Society states that you need to pull your penis out of the way to examine each testicle separately.

You then must hold one testicle between your thumbs and fingers with both hands. Next, roll the testicle gently between your fingers. You are doing this to see if you feel any hard lumps or nodules. Also check to see if there are any change in size, consistency, or shape.

Let the Doctor Feel Your (Easter Egg) Basket: You need to speak up if your physician is not being proactive about giving you a testicular exam with every check-up. I go to my doctor every three months and I am considering having him do an exam every time just to be sure. After all, I just turned thirty-nine and I am not getting any younger; I want to stay on top of my health as I age.

X-Rays & Ultrasounds: X-rays can be used to look for tumors on or around your testicles. But this is often used to see if the cancer has spread. There is another way to test for testicular cancer. If you or your doctor think there may be something that needs further examination of your testicles, an ultrasound can be ordered and can help doctors look for tumors that X-rays may not detect.

Testing the Testes: The doctor may want to run a blood test. The blood test will tell the doctor whether the cancer will remain in your body if the removal of your testicle is a solution.

Egg Replacements: The doctor might decide that you will need to have your testicle removed. The doctor can use a prosthetic, saline-filled testicle to replace the removed testicle if you choose. To remove lymph nodes your doctor would have to perform surgery. But caution: this can cause nerve damage and might make it difficult to ejaculate.

Radiation & Chemo: Doctors can use radiation to kill cancer cells. If your doctor has removed your testicle, this treatment might be used to ensure the removal of cancer cells. Please be aware that radiation treatment may cause nausea, fatigue, irritation of skin and reduction of sperm count. Chemotherapy may be also recommended by your doctor, before or after lymph nodes are removed. It often is used if the cancer has traveled to other parts of your body. Be aware that nausea, fatigue, hair loss and increased risk of other infections of the body may be side effects.

Preserve Your Yolk: Many of us want to have biological children. Talk to your doctor about sperm preservation before undergoing treatment. Also, let me state that I am the father of two adopted children, so sperm preservation is not your only option to be a parent.


Just*in Time: Why I Love Brian Sims' PrEP Post

Just*in Time

by Justin B. Terry-Smith

April 26, 2019

If anyone is in tune with politics (at least in the Mid-Atlantic region) you should know the name Brian Sims [A&U, September 2018]. Brian Sims is a Democratic Pennsylvania State Representative, and also a part of the LGBTQ community. Sims is very vocal on any and all social media outlets, whether on Twitter, where he states that he is a "civil rights attorney, College Football Captain, Bearded, RuPaul's Drag Race fanatic, and Little Mermaid enthusiast," or on his Instagram, where he has pictures from his day-to-day life with his dog, friends, and family.

One recent April post on Instagram received a lot of attention. Sims posted a picture of his daily pre-exposure prophylaxis (PrEP) stating, "PrEP/PEP: Starting this day off smart, proactive, and in control! Think this is an invite to talk about my sex life? It is not. Think it is an invite to shame me or anyone else? Grow up. 'Stigma' is the thing our enemies want us to be stunted by. It literally kills us. It is stupid and we control our own fate. No shame in this game. Just Pride. #PrEPsavesLIVES." Basically, with this post Brian Sims came out of the PrEP closet. When I saw this, I could not be prouder of Sims. So, this entry is dedicated to Rep. Sims for his courage and leadership. Here are five things about Sims' PrEP post that make the world better for HIV prevention.


**1. Lead by Example**
Sims is doing just that—leading by example. When most people in the general public see someone, who is well known within their own community adhere to preventative measures, it is more likely that they will conform to that same prevention method. It is important that the

LGBTQ community accept PrEP as a preventative measure but also know they can use condoms with or without PrEP.

## 2. Inexpensive PrEP Campaign

Sims basically made his own HIV prevention campaign for PrEP. Being a part of HIV campaigns, I can tell you firsthand that it is easy to be a model but not easy to create nor fund an HIV campaign. On Sims' Facebook page he posted a picture of his PrEP regimen and stated, "Starting this day off smart, proactive, and in control! How about you? #PrEPsavesLIVES." That line itself can be a PrEP campaign! With marketing and messaging it could be bigger than the as of now 3.1K liked post.

## 3. Fighting PrEP Stigma

Ever since PrEP became available it has faced criticism. People have said PrEP is nothing but an excuse for people to have "unprotected" sex. Well, as most of us know, PrEP is an HIV prophylaxis, which mean whoever is on PrEP and engaging in intercourse is indeed having protected sex, with or without a condom. Sims is taking a stand with his post in stating on his Facebook page by making sure people know the effects of stigma and proclaiming his pride.

## 4. Empowerment Is Everything

Empowering a population is hard work, but, with people like Sims, it becomes easier. Empowering a population to be able to take back their lives by giving them the power to choose what prophylaxis they want to use is paramount in HIV prevention. Empowering the LGBTQ population in HIV prevention needs to be at the forefront of any PrEP campaign because the LGBTQ community is one that is deeply affected by HIV.

## 5.Starting a Discussion

Looking at his page and reading the replies to his post, I was reminded that there are so many different sides to the question, "Should I go on PrEP?" I am guessing that Sims is not telling people what do to or how to lives their lives, but simply informing us what his HIV prevention path is. Since today the post has garnered over 530 comments and the replies are still increasing. There are people citing the negatives and positives about going on PrEP; people praising Sims for his courage (me included) and thanking him for his attempt at dismantling stigma. All in all, he started a discussion that will have legs.

I wanted to commend Brian Sims and say, "Thank you, sir. You are truly an amazing man and I am glad you have decided to do this. This takes chutzpah (guts) and there are a lot of people who are on PrEP who are shamed into the PrEP closet. You have made it easier for people to say, 'Yes, I am on PrEP and I'm proud of it.' You have made those people that have been already empowered by you to stand up for themselves in the face of adversity and take control of their own HIV prevention measure. Good on you, sir, and thank you again."

Just*in Time: HIV & Your Independence

**Just*in Time**

by Justin B. Terry-Smith

July is a good time to talk about HIV Independence Day.
Breaking up is hard to do for everyone. Even amicable breakups are hard. But picture this, you are living with HIV and you have finally found someone to love and to love you. Just like any other relationship you rely and depend on each other whether it be for physical, emotional, or financial support. There are certain things one must consider when going through a breakup while living with HIV. But the most important thing is taking care of you, despite the hurt that you are feeling and will continue to feel. Now is the time for your Independence Day. YOU CAN DO THIS!

**1. Talk to someone**

I went through a very bad breakup and closed everyone out of my life. I started making bad decisions because I did not have an outlet to help me with my mental health. If you are not mentally healthy, chances are you are not taking care of yourself physically, which is directly related to keeping your HIV in control and your T-cell count up.

**2. Phone a fucking friend**

Trust me, if your catch phrase after your breakup is "I'm fine," most of your true friends will know that that is a bunch of bullshit. You need to keep your friends close to you to be able to cry on their shoulders every once in a while. After my bad breakup, my friends reminded me that I needed to eat and take my meds; if it were not for them, I might have gotten sicker than I already was. If you do not know this already, HIV likes to stop us from eating and helps us forget to take care of ourselves.

### 3. Get out and exercise

You need to remain active. The more sedentary you stay; the better HIV has a chance to get the best of you. Of course, everyone wants to go through that dramatic "staying inside your house, don't take a shower, eat junk food and watching depressing movies breakup" phase. I did go through that phase myself, but I said to myself, "I Ain't Got Time For That." I pulled up my bootstraps and went for a three-mile run. I turned my pain into physical wellness and when living with HIV you wanted to physically keep your body in shape.

### 4. Set a reminder

When you become depressed and start thinking about other people and their issues, you spend less time thinking about yourself. You will forget to take your medication at times. But my suggestion to offset this is to create a reminder on your smartphone to take your medication. Almost everyone in the world has a smartphone but in case you do not write a damn note!

### 5. The way to get over someone is to get under a new one

Okay, this is not a solution and nor do I advise it. The best thing to do is to sometimes be by yourself. By being by yourself, it allows you to think and refocus. Since you have more time to yourself fill it up with something positive (pun intended). Get involved in the HIV community; you will find friends and a network to help you. You can be a part of an HIV awareness campaign, write a blog about HIV, etc.

The HIV community is very strong, and we need to be here to uplift each other. Most people who are living with HIV put a lot of emphasis on finding love. When they have not found love they think it is because of their HIV serostatus. What they really need to do is look in the mirror and love themselves before loving anyone else. A breakup always sucks, but we must celebrate our own Independence Day. Being independent, is one of the most empowering experiences in someone's life. Making the rules of life for yourself instead depending on someone to help make them for you can make someone take a long look at themselves as they become stronger and stronger. One must celebrate independence so they can help others celebrate their independence, too.

Just*in Time: 5 Simple Facts About HIV Remission & the London Patient
June 5, 2019

As the news came out about the London patient being cured of HIV, I thought of the whole question of HIV achieving remission. Just twelve years ago I remember hearing about Timothy Ray Brown, the Berlin patient (whom I know personally). The London patient and the Berlin patient were both cured by the same procedure. Both men had a bone marrow stem cell transplant to treat cancer. Both of the men got bone marrow from an HIV-resistant donor. Also, there is a third man from Dusseldorf, Germany, that had a similar bone marrow stem cell transplant to treat cancer and got bone marrow from an HIV-resistant donor. The Dusseldorf patient has been off his HIV medications for three months now but there is not enough time to say that this patient has been cured.

We should keep in mind what a "cure" means in the context of the everyday realities of people living with HIV/AIDS.

**5 Simple Facts about One Cure Approach for HIV**

1. It is super rare. Before both successful attempts to cure HIV there were many failed attempts in many patients. First the transplants from a HIV-resistant donor would be few and far between. Bone marrow transplants are also very risky; most doctors only perform this operation when there is a clinical reason, which would be cancer in these cases.

2. There must be a genetic match between the bone marrow donors and recipients. According to the U.S. Library of Science the C-C chemokine receptor type 5 (CCR5) is predicted to be a seven transmembrane protein similar to G protein-coupled receptors. This protein is articulated by T cells and macrophages and is known to be a significant co-receptor for macrophage-tropic virus, including HIV, to enter host cells. Defective alleles of this gene have been associated with the HIV infection resistance. Basically, both people involved in the operation have to have a matching CCR5 mutations.

3. CCR5 mutation is rare in itself. Professor Christopher Duncan told Science Daily that, "The fact that the CCR5-delta 32 mutation is restricted to Europe suggests that the plagues of the

Middle Ages played a big part in raising the frequency of the mutation. These plagues were also confined to Europe, persisted for more than 300 years and had a 100% case mortality." Basically, all people in that part of the world have a greater chance to have the match for the CCR5 that is HIV-resistant.

4. Americans not finding a cure of HIV could have something to do with it being the melting pot of the world. If there is a cure for HIV that could be found elsewhere other than in Europe, the United States has not found it yet. If it is hard for the Americans to find this cure, then we will need to generate more funding and more HIV research. The problem with that is the current Administration has halted certain HIV research, such as the study that would use fetal tissue to attempt to discover a cure for HIV. According to the Washington Post, the study was shut down because it uses fetal tissue implanted into mice.

5. Even though the HIV cure is rare, and I might not see one that I can take in my lifetime, it gives me hope for the future. It gives hope for the younger generation who are not really educated on the cure or HIV itself. Right now, HIV is something that some of us have to live with. I take one pill a day with food to suppress my HIV and that looks as if that is what I will have to do for the rest of my life, and I am okay with that. However, other people are not okay with that. No matter what, we need more funding for more HIV research; there has to be a cure out there for everyone, not just people from a certain part of the world. I still have hope.

Just*in Time: HIV & LGBTQ Domestic Violence
August 28, 2019

**Just*in Time**
by Justin B. Terry-Smith

Domestic violence is a serious threat to one's health whether it is mental, physical, emotional, or spiritual; throw HIV in the mix and it can be more and more disastrous. I have decided to write about same-sex intimate partner violence and HIV because these two subjects are very familiar to me, and I have been through both. I am a survivor of domestic abuse and I consider myself a survivor of HIV. The reason why I say I am a survivor of HIV is that I know plenty of my friends that, because of low self-esteem and HIV stigma, have died at very young ages. I chose not to let that happen to me and instead found the strength to live. We must use that same strength in order to be a survivor of domestic abuse. I recently had a very close and dear friend of mine go through a relationship that was physically, mentally, and emotionally abusive. He has finally cut his former abusive boyfriend out of his life and is now back in school, but it has been a long road for him to even get this far. My first piece of advice for victims of domestic abuse is to get away from your abuser. If, for whatever reason you cannot get away from your abuser, you can take steps to protect yourself.

**HIV Guilt** • I have seen it more than once. Boy meets boy, boy falls in love with boy, both boys become HIV-positive. In many cases like this, I see one who blames the other for acquiring HIV when neither knows for sure how it happened. And it should not matter if both consented to an open relationship. It is best if we blame the virus itself rather than ourselves. And unfortunately, I have seen this resentment led to physical and verbal abuse.

**Taking Away HIV Medication** • Abusive partners may try to cut you off from your HV resources. This is their way of manipulating you into staying with them. They might hide your medication or keep it from you so they can control when and how you take your medication. This is hard to get around. For reasons that have nothing to do with abuse, I sometimes keep a surplus of medication for emergencies and I have been separated from my medication. A solution might be that you can order more medication; however, make sure that your doctor knows that you need the medication to come to a different address and location, if you reside with your partner.

**Social Media** • Abusers like to make you think that they are reading your mind. My friend who I mentioned above had his Facebook account hacked by his abuser. The abuser saw all of our messages and began to try to guilt my friend based on what he learned. I told my friend to find shelter and the abuser grabbed screen shots of all of our messages and posted it to my friend's Facebook. He did that to try to show people how I and other friends were not good-hearted. But it only made him look more and more controlling. He could have taken it further and announced my friend's sexual orientation or HIV status, but he did not. I say this as a warning; change your passwords on all social media accounts and on all electronic devices. DO NOT GIVE ABUSERS ACCESS.

**HIV & Stress & Trauma** • Stress has been known to be directly related to one's HIV health, or health in general. When a person is living with HIV, stress affects one's T-cell count to the point where one's immune system is weakened. Trauma, such as experienced by individuals in an abusive relationship, is also a danger. According to the San Francisco AIDS Foundation's article, "What hard times & stress do for your HIV health," by Emily Land, MA, "Trauma significantly predicted risk of death from HIV or other causes. For everyone experience of trauma, risk of death increased by 17% and risk of HIV-related death increased by 22%. When three traumas were experienced, risk of death by any cause increased by 60% and HIV-related death by 83%."

**Money** • The abuser might hold money over the victim. For example, the abuser might tell the victim that they will take care of their victim by paying for their HIV medication. My friend would occasionally ask for money from me and I had no issue giving it to him because it might help him pay for food (which is vital for taking HIV medication). His abuser sent me a Facebook message and said, "I can't believe you are helping him pay for food when I provide for him." Of course, this is a form of control. I said to myself, "Well if he keeps asking me for money, how is it that you can say you provide for him". Then on social media the abuser paid for an $800 dog for his victim. So, I said something does not add up here. The abuser was withholding money from the victim, which he also needs for food and HIV medication.

I am going to leave you with some statistics about LGBTQ domestic violence. The CDC's National Intimate Partner and Sexual Violence Survey found for LGBTQ people: Forty-four percent of lesbians and sixty-one percent of bisexual women experience rape, physical violence, or stalking by an intimate partner, compared to thirty-five percent of heterosexual women. Twenty-six percent of gay men and thirty-seven percent of bisexual men experience rape, physical violence, or stalking by an intimate partner, compared to twenty-nine percent of heterosexual men. Forty-six percent of bisexual women have been raped, compared to seventeen percent of heterosexual women and thirteen percent of lesbians. Twenty-two percent of bisexual women have been raped by an intimate partner, compared to nine percent of heterosexual women. Forty percent of gay men and forty-seven percent of bisexual men have experienced sexual violence other than rape, compared to twenty-one percent of heterosexual men. You are not alone! If you are being abused, I encourage you to seek counseling and leave the situation as soon as possible. You might need to stay at a shelter or halfway house; look for a place that is LGBTQ and HIV-friendly. There are certain centers that focus on the LGBTQ community that provide food (which is a need for most HIV medications), shelter, job training, and education resources, as well.

Just*in Time: Honoring the Pathbreakers
September 14, 2019

**Just*in Time**

by Justin B. Terry-Smith

Being an HIV activist is a labor of love. One of the things that I hear a lot from the older generation of HIV activists is that I will never know how it feels to go to funerals every week and they are right. I was not there, and it is not anyone's fault; I was not born until 1979, after all. But I have never forgotten that generation that endured the atrocities of HIV/AIDS in the 1980s and 1990s. Here are five ways that I pay homage to the people that HIV/AIDS directly affected.

**Visit the AIDS Memorial Quilt**

A little history about the Quilt is that it was created in November 1985 by activist Cleve Jones. While planning the 1985 march to honor San Francisco Supervisor Harvey Milk and Mayor George Moscone, who were assassinated while in office, Jones learned that over 1,000 San Franciscans had been lost to AIDS. He asked the marchers to make a placard of a friend or loved who had died of AIDS-related causes. Jones and others climbed onto ladders to tape these placards to the walls of the San Francisco Federal Building. The placards of names resembled a quilt and Cleve and others thought to make this project bigger. Jones created the first panel for the AIDS Memorial Quilt in memory of his friend Marvin Feldman. Jones and Mike Smith formally organized the NAMES Project Foundation. The AIDS Memorial Quilt is always on display somewhere on December 1, which is World AIDS Day. It is now so large that it is broken up to be viewed.

**Listen to a Survivor's Story**

Make time to sit down with a long-term survivor to listen to their story. Ask them as many questions as it takes to fully understand and grasp their experience. Even if you were not alive at that point in time or you were not in touch with the community, it does not mean you cannot empathize. There are some survivors that will say to you, "You will never understand what it means to be living in a time period where all your friends are dying or dead." This is true. But when I hear this, I remember that I had my own struggles with my group of friends who I grew up with. Half of them are dead because of HIV denial. Everyone has their own story, and it is important to listen to the past so you can move forward into the future.

**Look Up the Deceased**

When I learned of my own positive status, I became curious about the history of HIV/AIDS. A big part of that is how AIDS came into the mainstream consciousness. One of those ways was that, when heterosexuals and famous people started acquiring HIV in greater numbers, more and more people started paying more attention. I researched Rock Hudson, Gia Marie Carangi, Alison Gertz, among others. The more I researched people from the past the more I was able to get a glimpse into their lives. It also allowed me to look within myself and ask, "Justin, what impression do you want to leave the world and how will it help others?"

**Research the Origins of HIV/AIDS**

Being an HIV/STI Advice Columnist I get this question all the time: "Where did AIDS come from?" This is a loaded question because there are multiple theories. What I would most concern myself with is finding out how it came into the human population and what theory am I going to believe as truth. That is what I would tell all of you. If you do not believe me and my advice, at least believe in something.

**Respect Your Elders**

I will be the first to admit that I do not get along with everyone, but I try my best to respect those who came before me in this battle to stop HIV/AIDS. I respect them by telling my own story, of how I acquired HIV and how I am living with the virus. Now, I ask you to do something to help your elders who are long-term HIV survivors. Join a charity, work at an LGBTQ elderly home that might specifically focus on LGBTQ individuals with HIV/AIDS, befriend a person who lived through the AIDS epidemic in the 1980s and 1990s. Come up with your own and email me with what you did!

*All names have been changed to protect the identities of all who have asked Justin for advice.

CPSIA information can be obtained
at www.ICGtesting.com
Printed in the USA
BVHW092214230321
603261BV00014B/1108